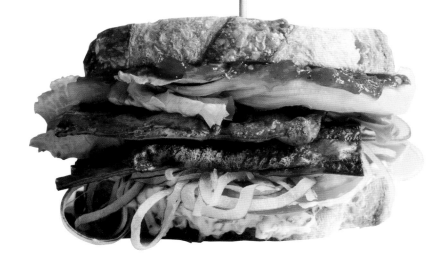

THE WICKED

FREE.
FROM.
ANIMALS.

HEALTHY

COOKBOOK

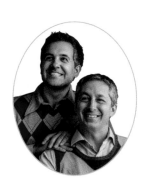

CHAD SARNO, DEREK SARNO, AND DAVID JOACHIM

Foreword by **WOODY HARRELSON**

Photographs by **EVA KOSMAS FLORES**

sphere

SPHERE

3 5 7 9 10 8 6 4 2

First published in the United States in 2018 by Grand
Central Life & Style, an imprint of Grand Central
Publishing.

First published in Great Britain in 2018 by Sphere

A CIP catalogue record for this book is available from the
British Library.

ISBN: 978-0-7515-7283-4

Printed and bound in Italy by L.E.G.O S.p.A

Recipe for Tal Ronnen's Eggless Pasta Dough on page
208 excerpted from Crossroads copyright © 2015 by
TRB Management, LLC. Used by permission of Artisan,
a division of Workman Publishing Co., Inc., New York.
All Rights Reserved.

Print book interior design by Toni Tajima.

Papers used by Sphere are from well-managed forests and
other responsible sources.

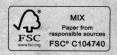

Sphere
An imprint of Little, Brown Book Group
Carmelite House
50 Victoria Embankment
London EC4Y 0DZ

An Hachette UK Company
www.hachette.co.uk

www.littlebrown.co.uk

A note to UK readers: To help with popular US terms and
ingredients, you will find some tips on page 296.

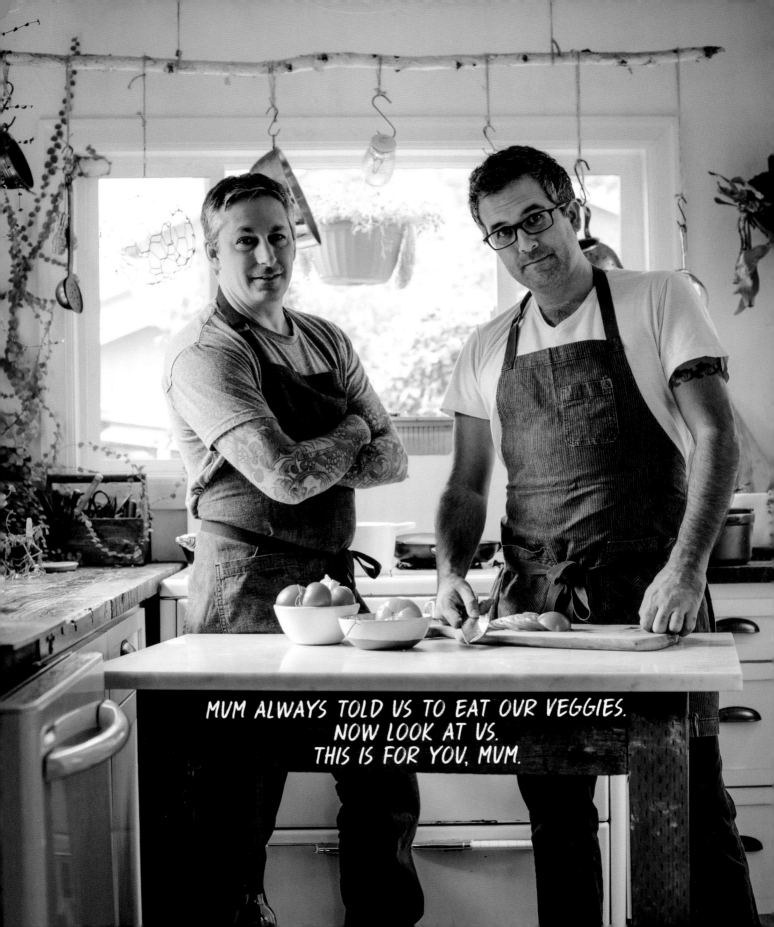

MUM ALWAYS TOLD US TO EAT OUR VEGGIES.
NOW LOOK AT US.
THIS IS FOR YOU, MUM.

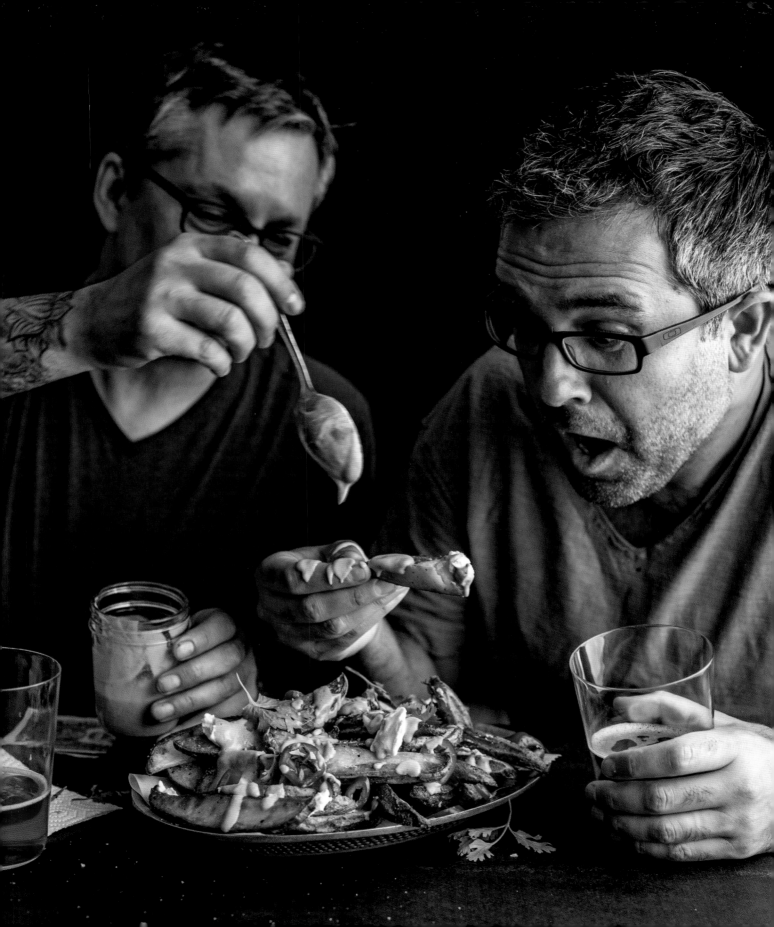

CONTENTS

RECIPE LIST

FOREWORD

I've been eating vegan for more than thirty years. To me, plant-based just seems like the right way to eat—for a healthy body and a healthy planet. When I'm working, I eat super clean. I go almost fully raw. It makes my mind sharper, helps me focus, and no after-lunch slow down.

This is the kind of food that Chad Sarno made for me all the time when I was preparing for movie roles. Chad was my personal chef for a bunch of films. I've tasted Chad's food day in and day out, in different seasons, at home, on movie sets, and around the world. It's all freakin' delicious. Over the years, I've also gotten to know Chad's brother, Derek, and together in the kitchen, these two guys are the Dream Team!

Chad and Derek are doing some incredible work. They are at the forefront of a plant-based food movement that's been building for decades and is now becoming a tsunami. Even if you know nothing about cooking, these guys will teach you how to make your meals taste amazing. Like their chapter title says, healthy food doesn't have to taste like shit. And they show you how to have fun in the kitchen! But the best thing? The recipes are *not* just for committed vegans. This food is for everybody. It is just good, sexy food anyone would love.

This whole book is basically the blueprint for treating yourself right, enjoying everything you eat, and having a positive impact on the world around you. Now there are no more excuses. Go ahead and indulge in the absolute best-tasting and most life-affirming food on the planet.

—WOODY HARRELSON, award-winning actor and food activist

INTRODUCTION

Diet, Schmiet

Here's the deal: We're chefs and brothers (secretly, ninjas) and though we come from two different professional backgrounds, we found common ground in the Wicked Healthy culinary arts. We're from New England, so for us, "Wicked Healthy" means "good-for-you food that tastes so good you think it must be bad for you." The bottom line is, we want you to be healthy because healthy people are full of life. They're upbeat, confident, and energetic. We want you to eat more vegetables. Especially the green ones! We'd prefer it if they were organic and maybe even local. Most importantly, we want them to taste great. Go easy on added sugars, saturated fats, and salt. Eat lots of fruit. Make an effort to move around every day. And use your freakin' brain. Stay on the Wicked Healthy path and understand that you're going to wander off the trail and go out to eat now and then—just maybe think for a second before ordering.

As professional chefs, we have owned and opened restaurants all over the world. We also worked as global chefs at Whole Foods Market and currently teach students around the world about healthy cooking. Over the years, we've collaborated with all sorts of doctors and nutritionists. They all say the same thing: Eat more vegetables, fruits, nuts, beans, and whole grains. Yeah, yeah. Everybody hears that, right? So what are we bringing to the table? What can we do for you? We can show you incredible new ways to actually enjoy all these foods. We know from experience that healthy eating is not about starvation or choking down food that tastes like shit. It's about celebrating what tastes great in the world of plants. Stuffed Avocado Bar (page 221) to share with friends? Bring it on.

Chocoholic Fudge Brownies with Sea Salt and Dried Strawberries (page 238)? Now we're talkin'. Avocados and chocolate are good for you. Eat them! We're all about celebrating what you should be eating, not shunning what you shouldn't. We're plant pushers, not meat shamers! Face it, we all indulge in our own vices on occasion—whatever diet we follow—and that's just fine.

Our overall food philosophy is simple: shoot for 80% healthy and 20% wicked and you'll be 100% sexy. Maybe that means eating healthy during the week, then loosening up on the weekends. Or maybe you stay healthy during the day then get wicked at dinner now and then. You have to figure out exactly what kind of 80/20 approach works best for you. The Wicked Healthy path is not about strict

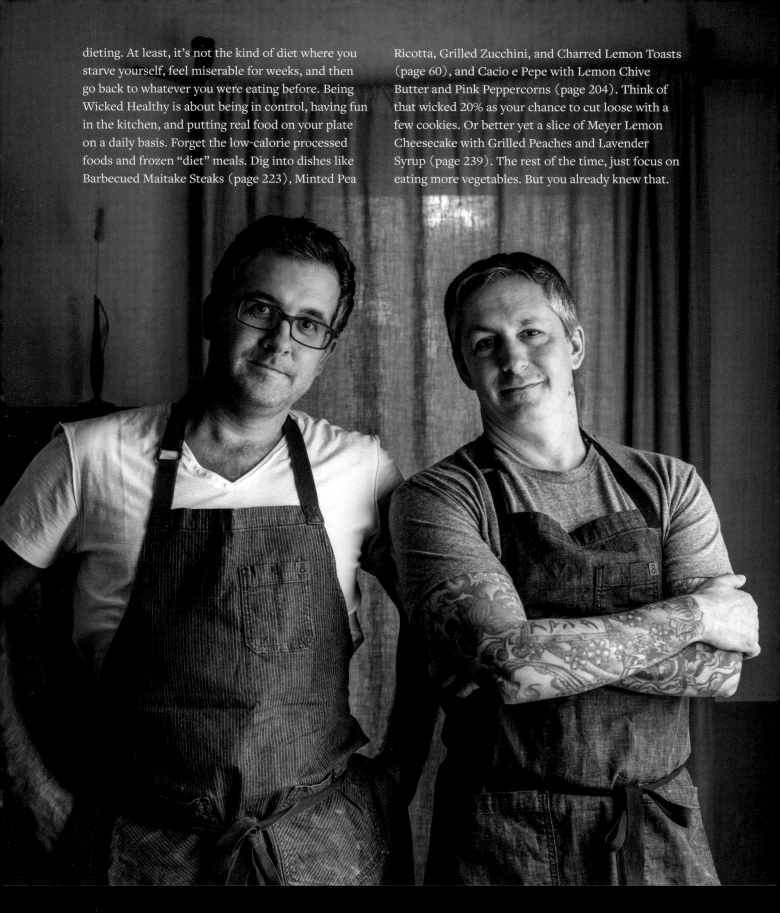

dieting. At least, it's not the kind of diet where you starve yourself, feel miserable for weeks, and then go back to whatever you were eating before. Being Wicked Healthy is about being in control, having fun in the kitchen, and putting real food on your plate on a daily basis. Forget the low-calorie processed foods and frozen "diet" meals. Dig into dishes like Barbecued Maitake Steaks (page 223), Minted Pea Ricotta, Grilled Zucchini, and Charred Lemon Toasts (page 60), and Cacio e Pepe with Lemon Chive Butter and Pink Peppercorns (page 204). Think of that wicked 20% as your chance to cut loose with a few cookies. Or better yet a slice of Meyer Lemon Cheesecake with Grilled Peaches and Lavender Syrup (page 239). The rest of the time, just focus on eating more vegetables. But you already knew that.

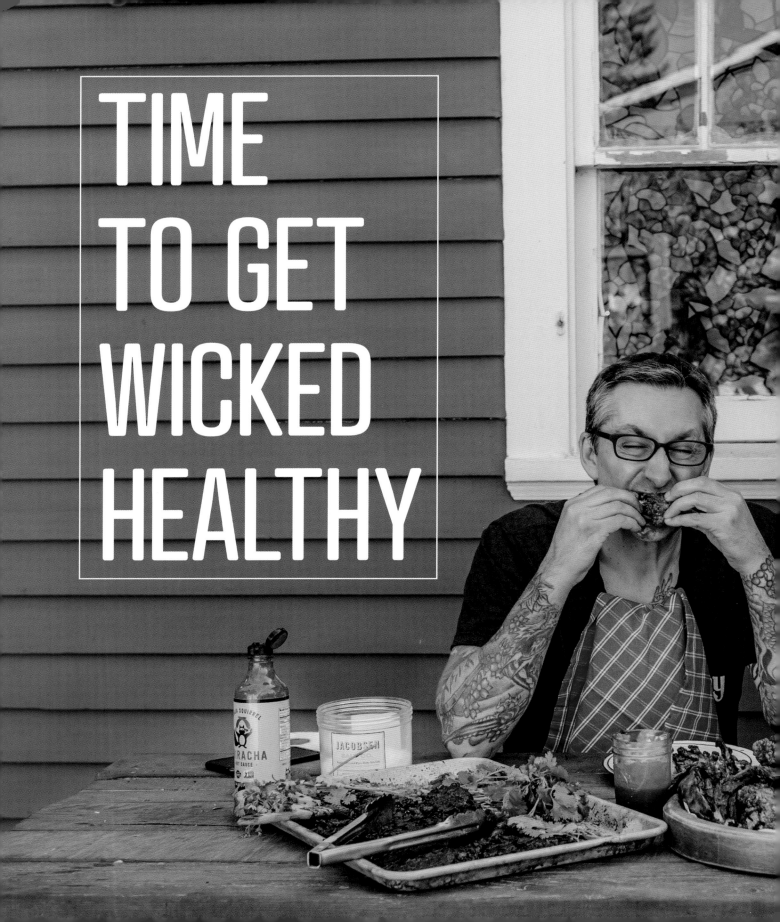

TIME TO GET WICKED HEALTHY

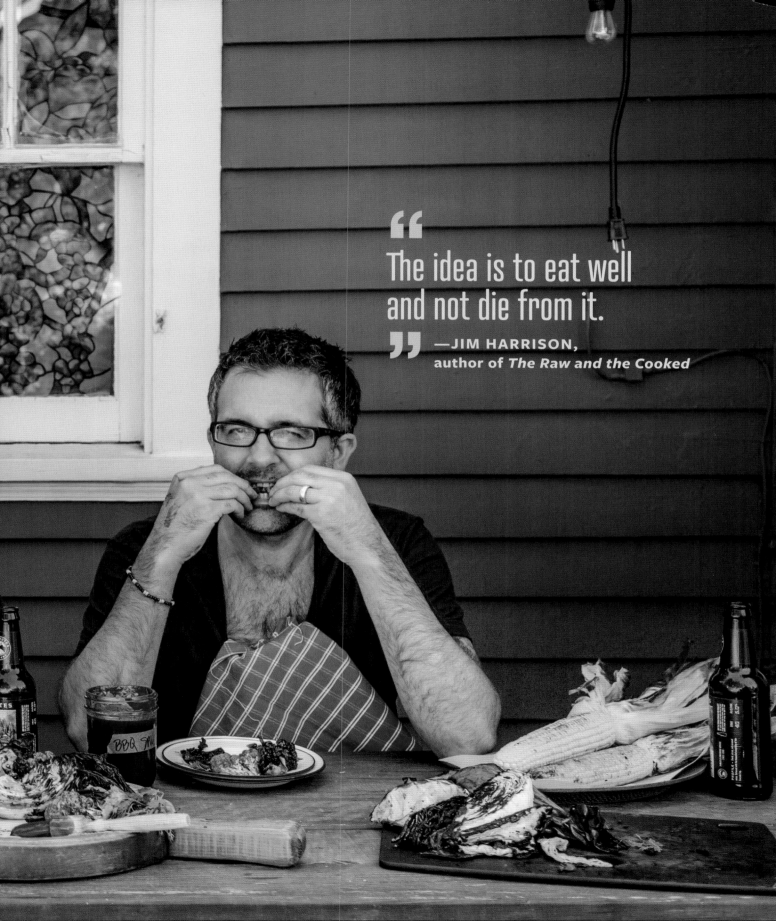

"The idea is to eat well and not die from it.

—JIM HARRISON, author of *The Raw and the Cooked*

NUTRITION IS CONFUSING. IT'S COMPLEX.

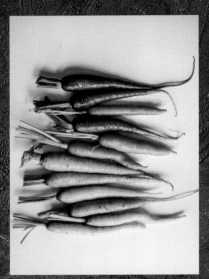

The good news is that all the health experts—no matter what "diet" they promote—say the same thing: Everyone should eat more plant foods and less processed foods. More real food and fewer packaged food "products." More sweet potatoes and fewer bags of sweet potato chips. The naked truth is that we are overfed and undernourished—particularly in industrialized countries. We just need to eat more whole fruits, vegetables, nuts, seeds, beans, lentils, and whole grains. Scientists have discovered that plants can help protect us against everything from Alzheimer's and diabetes to heart disease and many cancers. There's even some research showing that plant protein can keep you feeling full longer than animal protein, which may help prevent overeating. Researchers have also found that eating more plant foods can help improve everything from our body weight and eyesight to our skin and gut health. Think about it. Almost all preventative and healing medicines are made from plants. Why not just eat the plants themselves?

Wicked Healthy is a commonsense approach to health. Everybody knows we should eat more plant foods. It's better for us. It's better for the planet. The problem is, we're just not used to doing it, and most of us don't have the kitchen *smahhts* to make these foods taste their best. We're used to reaching for a bag of Doritos, not a handful of almonds. At some point in your life, you realize you gotta take care of yourself. It's hard to change. However, when you eat something really delicious that also happens to be real food, that experience alone can inspire you to eat better.

Maybe you think healthy food can't be delicious. This is where Wicked Healthy flips the conversation. Just because it's plant-based doesn't mean it doesn't taste good. We are chefs. We've spent decades practicing and perfecting our craft, making all sorts of plant foods taste great. You've heard that "an apple a day keeps the doctor away." We're here to show you the 2.0 of that concept. We're drizzling that apple with Mango Sriracha Caramel (page 270) to make it irresistibly good. We're caramelizing that apple in a hot pan and adding it to a bowl of oatmeal for a comfort-food breakfast. We've got a lot of

> ❝ There is absolutely no nutrient, no protein, no vitamin, no mineral—no nothing—found in meats and dairy products that you cannot obtain from a plant-based food. ❞
>
> —MICHAEL KLAPER, MD

tricks up our sleeves. Thinking like a chef also means getting yourself organized in the kitchen. A well-stocked pantry and a few pro-cook habits can make cooking a breeze, not a chore. Ever hear of batch cooking? If you're making rice, beans, or noodles on the weekend, make a double batch so you have some for quick meals later in the week. If you're making Wicked Healthy Cheese Sauce for Mac & Cheese (page 260), blend up a couple of quarts and keep the sauce in the fridge for a week of different dishes like Smoky Poutine (page 72) and Sweet Potato Gratin with Crispy Onions and Rosemary (page 185).

The Wicked Healthy approach is all about the food. Put down that bag of potato chips for a second and get your ass in the kitchen. Take control of what you put in your body. We'll show you how to build flavor with some basic—and not-so-basic—techniques. Did you know that searing and browning food actually create new flavors that weren't there before? That's why grilled food tastes so awesome! A more personal question: Do you shave your vegetables? You should! If you don't already have a mandoline (vegetable shaver), pick up a cheap handheld one so you can cut radishes, asparagus, cucumbers, and other vegetables wicked thin, wicked fast. Shaving vegetables makes it soooo easy to put together a crunchy fresh salad. We also developed this really cool press-and-sear technique that intensifies the taste and texture of mushrooms. It makes them super dense and meaty. Check it out on page 42.

EAT PLANTS, GET HEALTHY

Eating more plants is a simple dietary approach endorsed by every doctor and health organization in the world. We like to focus on making plants taste wicked delicious. But here's how the health experts get the point across.

"The basic principles of good diets are so simple that I can summarize them in just ten words: *Eat less, move more, eat lots of fruits and vegetables.*"

—MARION NESTLE, award-winning professor of nutrition at New York University, *What to Eat* (North Point Press, 2006)

"Eat food. Not too much. Mostly plants."

—MICHAEL POLLAN, award-winning author and professor of journalism at the University of California, Berkeley, *In Defense of Food* (Penguin Press, 2008)

"Eat a healthy diet with an emphasis on plant foods. Choose foods and drinks in amounts that help you get to and maintain a healthy weight. Limit how much processed meat and red meat you eat. Eat at least 2½ cups of vegetables and fruits each day. Choose whole grains instead of refined grain products."

—AMERICAN CANCER SOCIETY, *Summary of Guidelines on Nutrition and Physical Activity,* June 2016

"A healthy eating pattern includes a variety of vegetables from all of the subgroups—dark green, red and orange, legumes (beans and peas), starchy, and other; fruits, especially whole fruits; grains, at least half of which are whole grains; fat-free or low-fat dairy, including milk, yogurt, cheese, and/or fortified soy beverages; a variety of protein foods, including seafood, lean meats and poultry, eggs, legumes (beans and peas), and nuts, seeds, and soy products; and oils."

—*2015–2020 Dietary Guidelines for Americans,* U.S. Departments of Health and Human Services (HHS) and Agriculture (USDA), Key Recommendations

THIS WILL BE THE BEST $20 YOU EVER SPENT!

80% *Healthy* + 20% *Wicked* = 100% *Sexy*

Before we geek out on you with more chef talk, we have to say that following the Wicked Healthy path will help you no matter what special diet you're on. As chefs and brothers, we've spent (collectively) more than 30 years consulting with various doctors, nutritionists, retailers, food manufacturers, restaurants, students, and clients about diets ranging from macrobiotic and diabetic to gluten-free, low-carb, no-added-sugar and no-added-oil. Over the years, we combined the expert advice of numerous respected health professionals with the concerns and tastes of busy home cooks just like you. Then we rolled it all together. That's how we came up with our formula: 80% healthy + 20% wicked = 100% sexy.

Simply put, that means we should eat healthy foods 80% of the time. We all know what the healthy foods are: whole, unprocessed plant foods! Explore the thousands of vegetables, fruits, nuts, seeds, beans, whole grains, herbs, flowers, and mushrooms out there. Try new ones and find the ones that taste good to you. Use the recipes and ideas in this book to make them even more delicious. The other 20% of the time, give yourself a break. Get wicked. Indulge— whatever that may mean to you. Go ahead and give yourself that 20% of latitude. That way, you're more likely to stick with your overall eating goals.

How do we stay Wicked Healthy? We'll admit it straight up: We do not plan all our meals for every day of the week. And not every meal is low-calorie or packed with superfoods. We're chefs. We love to get inspired by ingredients and flavor. Texture! Temperature! Aroma! So maybe today we indulged a bit too much. Tomorrow we'll eat healthy. No problem. It's all good. It's all about finding the balance that works for you. We had a client call us once because she "fell off the wagon" and ate a handful of cookies. "What have I done?" she cried into the phone. "It's okay!" we told her. Eating a couple of cookies is not a big deal. Now, eating the whole bag while sitting on the couch and watching TV soap operas...day after day...that's not so good. Maybe it's time to get out of the house.

We will never tell you *not* to eat certain foods. We're plant pushers, pure and simple. Wicked Healthy is here to show you all the great food you could be eating when you put plants at the center of your diet. Like our Avocado Toasts with Radishes and Meyer Lemon (page 58). So friggin' good. Orecchiette with Grilled Squash, Preserved

> **When you eat healthfully, your body gravitates relatively rapidly toward a better weight.**
> —JOEL FUHRMAN, MD

Lemon, and Herbs (page 205). Yum. Grilled Almond Butter, Chocolate, and Raspberry Sandwich (page 136). Bring it!

You have to figure out exactly how the 80/20 approach fits into your lifestyle. Maybe it means you eat healthy Monday to Friday, then Saturday and Sunday you party like a rock star. Or maybe you just try to eat a healthy breakfast and lunch every day, then indulge at dinner. Angel by day, devil by night. Or maybe you like to get really focused and go for 80% healthy and 20% wicked at each meal, like having a breakfast bowl of oatmeal with cranberries and pecans (all healthy), then topping it with a drizzle of rich coconut cream and warm maple syrup (both wicked). That works, too. Just keep it 80/20. No matter how you divide it up—by week, day, or meal—**if you stick with it and eat 80% healthy, those good-for-you foods will start to edge out the less healthy foods you were eating before.** As your palate adjusts, you should find that your cravings for salty, fatty, sugary junk food start to fade. You should also start to feel good about what's going on in your body—especially if you had been feeling low energy or struggling with your weight. When you're on the Wicked Healthy path, you will start feeling better and more confident, and have more energy. That vitality alone will make you look and feel 100% sexy inside and out.

No matter what your health goals are, even if you're following strict doctor's orders for a specific health condition, you'll find 150 inventive recipes here to keep you satisfied. We make it real easy by indexing all the special diet recipes, starting on page 287. Doc told you to cut back on sugar? Go check out the list of no-sugar-added recipes. Gluten-free? No problem. Heading into a dry January cleanse? We have a list of recipes for that, too. We found the missing link between the doctor's orders and a delicious meal on your table. Our Spicy Coconut–Corn Crack (page 158) has no added oils, limited sugars, and minimal salt. It's also wicked good because we know how to make food taste amazing without always reaching for the processed oils and sugars. That Wicked Healthy Cheese Sauce we mentioned earlier? It's gluten-free, oil-free, and added-sugar-free. And we could eat it every damn day of the week.

> **One of the main causes of death is fretting about your diet.**
> —JIM HARRISON,
> author of *A Really Big Lunch*

Our recipes range from quick and easy everyday meals to fancier dishes for special meals with friends and family. None of it is "diet" food. Forget the idea that good-for-you food tastes like shit. It's all freaking delicious and you don't need tweezers to make a sexy meal. Two things guide all our recipes: flavor and plants. We like to pack in as much of both as possible. We're talking about everything from simple Potato and Cauliflower Bisque (page 157) to warm you up on a chilly winter night, to a nice plated dish of

> **Approximately 70% of the calories consumed on the standard American diet come from the same ingredients used to make doughnuts (added oils, sweeteners, and refined flours). Whatever diet you decide to follow, at the very least, please be sure you are not eating doughnuts for two out of every three meals per day!** —ALONA PULDE, MD, AND MATTHEW LEDERMAN, MD

Spring Agnolotti with Favas, Mint, and Sherry Cream (page 214) for that special someone you're having over for dinner.

Don't get bogged down in all the nutrition confusion. **Take the keys and get your ass in the driver's seat of your own health.** Keep it simple and have fun with your food. There's nothing wrong with spending a little time to prepare dinner. It's part of the commitment you should make to treat yourself right. Hang out in the kitchen and enjoy making good food for yourself, your family, and your friends. Just aim to eat 80% healthy and 20% wicked, and you'll feel 100% sexy inside and out.

How Did We Get Here?

You can take the boys out of New England, but you can't take New England out of the boys. That means we still have the same can-do, wise-ass attitude we had as kids growing up in New Hampshaah. We love taking risks and solving problems—especially if it means we get to play with food. Our family was a huge influence on us, foodwise. We cooked with our nana and mom all the time. Nana always had something on the stove, from her signature red sauce (page 265) to traditional Italian dishes like manicotti. At one point, Mom dove into Cantonese cooking and turned us on to the pleasures of stir-fries, dumplings, and bamboo steam baskets, which we still can't get enough of. In high school, we both ended up taking kitchen jobs. From there, we went our separate ways to refine our craft and passions. Eventually, though, we ended up back in the kitchen together making Wicked Healthy food.

Wicked Healthy took root on a farm in Maine sometime in 2003/2004. Inspired by Helen and Scott Nearing's book, *The Good Life,* Derek started the South Hill Farm project. As a chef, he wanted to go to the source and see where his food came from, and how it was grown. He planted 350 tomato plants, 100 blueberry bushes, and rows and rows of potatoes, salad greens, and herbs. Chad was living in Maine at the time and we started cooking together

In high school, I was a pretty good kid, but my senior year, I had zero fucks to give and was still dealing with the sudden losses of close family members and my best friend. After graduation, I reluctantly went to culinary school in Rhode Island. There, I learned how to drink beer and make a roux. Let's be honest.

I began cooking professionally at a place called Lucas's Greenhouse in Hampton Falls, New Hampshire. The head chef, Skip, took me under his wing for four years and taught me more than any school ever could. I worked with some talented people in restaurants up and down the East Coast, from Massachusetts to Maine, at ski resorts, and even on a lobster boat off Little Cranberry Island, Maine, for four seasons.

In 1999, my son Jake was born and that lit a fire under my ass. I struck out on my own and opened a slew of restaurants and catering companies in New England, including Mahalos Catering, the One Hundred Club, and Mizuna. I also gave organic farming a shot. I wanted to learn more about good ingredients, where they come from, and how to grow them. Our catering kitchens were located on the Seacoast of New Hampshire, and we handled big and small events for corporate executives with a focus on private jets and parties. Even back in 2005, we had prepared dinners to go and e-commerce meal services, and we catered big movie premieres like *The Da Vinci Code* and *Angels and Demons*. I'm very grateful to the Browns for introducing me to the Buddhist monastery I would later enter into when I sold my businesses and went off the grid.

—DEREK

After high school, it became clear that I had to leave our small town in New England and explore the world. I went to college in the sticks of Colorado to figure out life. That's where one of my closest friends, Michael, passed away suddenly on a hiking trip, which shook me to the core and propelled me to do some soul searching. I left school and started hitchhiking around the country, looking for a deeper purpose in life. I spent a ton of time camping, foraging for food, taking kitchen jobs for cash, and living like a nomad. I completely immersed myself in the world of clean eating and animal rights and had the passion to learn and hone my kitchen skills. I had already been following a plant-based diet due to asthma. Yes, I was the lucky kid dependent on inhalers to get him through the day. Fortunately, in my teen years, a family friend suggested cutting out dairy products, and after trying it for a few months, my asthma subsided. That one simple dietary change schooled me on the fact that food has a tremendously powerful effect on your health. That experience carved my path ahead. From that point forward, I was a sponge, learning all I could about the food-health connection and teaching it to anyone who would listen.

I eventually wound up cooking at Breitenbush Hot Springs, a plant-based retreat center in the middle of the Willamette National Forest in Oregon. By the end of the 1990s, I took a position as staff chef at Living Light Culinary Arts Institute, a small raw-food culinary school in northern California. That job propelled me deep into the plant-based and raw-food communities.

Fast-forward a few years, and I found myself in Maui, where my dad and our other brother, Darren, lived. While beach camping and exploring the island, some crazy good fortune struck and a woman named Laura, now a close friend, picked me up. I found out later that Laura's partner was Woody Harrelson. After this chance meeting, I worked with Woody and his family for several years as their personal chef on a number of film sets.

In 2005, my daughter, Amaya, was born, and then came four whirlwind years opening plant-based SAF (simple authentic food) restaurants and living in Europe. I was bouncing to a different restaurant every couple of weeks—from three SAF locations in Istanbul to one in Munich to another two locations opening in London. Business was booming.

—*CHAD*

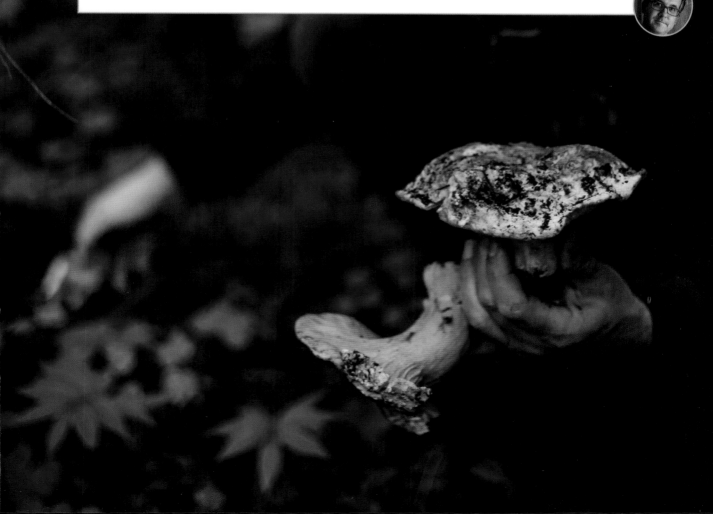

at the farm. It was rocky at first. We figured it out as we went. We had been going our separate ways for more than ten years, and although we were brothers, we were very different cooks. One of us had a backpack full of sprouting equipment and the other had a classic French mandoline. We made fun of each other in the kitchen—and still do. Secretly, though, each of us wanted to know more about what the other was doing. We cooked together at a couple of food events and combined our passion for local foods, clean ingredients, and smart techniques. That's when the seeds of Wicked Healthy were sown.

During that time, there was a lot of growth, change, and excitement. Derek had just met the love of his life, Amanda, and they were engaged. Chad's daughter, Amaya, was born, and he was opening plant-based restaurants around the globe. A bright future was unfolding for both of us.

Then the unthinkable happened. Amanda was killed in a horrible car accident.

When Amanda died, my world was shattered with the sudden loss of my fiancée. It's incredibly hard to convey the feeling. Life became so precious and I didn't ever want anyone to feel that kind of anguish. All this time what I had thought of as being a success was just ego-driven and a distraction from real purpose in life.

I ended up going off the radar and entered Padma Samye Ling, a Tibetan Buddhist monastery in upstate New York. I needed space to rebuild my life, and it was the only thing that made sense at the time. It was either that or self-destruction. I had always been into martial arts and dabbled in meditation. The monastery just accelerated the meditation side of things. I learned to simply sit, meditate, and practice compassion for others and myself. I still practice today.

With some effort, I started cooking again, diving deep into the monastery teachings, learning as much as I could and practicing mindfulness. It gradually became clear that, as a cook, I had the ability—and the responsibility—to nourish others. I became very conscious of what I was putting into other people's bodies and started cooking with greater intention. I didn't talk with any doctors. I didn't read any cookbooks. It was just obvious that the most beneficial way to feed people was with plant-based, life-supporting food. To me, it's common sense—not an ego thing! Animals should not have to suffer just to feed our indulgences. I focused on preparing meals with a strengthened intention of feeding people delicious, nourishing food that promoted life beyond just our taste buds.

—DEREK

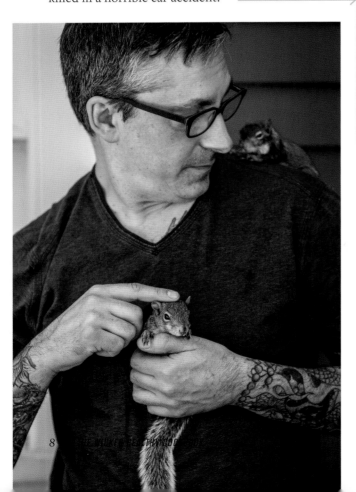

By early 2010, Derek had joined Whole Foods Market as global healthy eating chef. Chad was already working at Whole Foods, and this is when Wicked Healthy really blossomed. Our job was to find common ground between the rock-solid health advice of Whole Foods Market's medical advisors and the busy schedules of everyday working people. We knew that people weren't willing to sacrifice flavor for health. They wouldn't just ditch their beloved burgers and suddenly start eating kale salads. We had to meet them halfway, to start with plant-based comfort foods like Margherita Pizza (page 99) and Mac & Cheese (page 261) and gradually incorporate more and more plants into their meals.

That's Wicked Healthy in a nutshell. It's an approach that anyone can take regardless of where you are with your healthy eating goals. We're all about showing you how to make good-for-you, plant-based food that tastes so friggin' delicious you think it must be bad for you.

> While Derek was in the monastery, I was opening an SAF restaurant in London, and after years of frantic openings, I was ready for a change. A dear friend, Benay, recommended the restaurant to John Mackey, the CEO of Whole Foods Market. John came in for dinner and we connected immediately over our shared passion for pushing plants. He mentioned his company's "core value of healthy eating," adding that maybe we could work together someday. I pursued that opportunity relentlessly and was eventually hired as the global coordinator of healthy eating at Whole Foods. I jumped into the role to co-create and launch the company's Healthy Eating Program for employees and customers. I have been an activist at heart for years, and this was the next step I was praying for—an opportunity to reach a wider audience with the plant-based message and be of greater benefit to the animals and the planet.
>
> My role at Whole Foods evolved to include recipe development and media work as the company's spokesperson for Healthy Eating and Culinary Education. As we refined the program and rolled it out, I worked closely with our medical advisory board, which included superstar doctors of the healthy eating world. This work later became branded as Health Starts Here, the global healthy eating program at Whole Foods Market.
>
> Around this time, I suggested to Derek that he leave the monastery and come back out into the world. He was cooking incredible plant-based food and had so much to share. I thought to myself, "Wouldn't it be amazing if we could work together? This is when the seeds of Wicked Healthy started to grow."

— CHAD

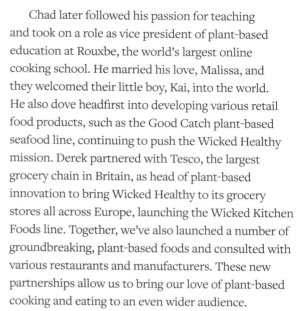

Chad later followed his passion for teaching and took on a role as vice president of plant-based education at Rouxbe, the world's largest online cooking school. He married his love, Malissa, and they welcomed their little boy, Kai, into the world. He also dove headfirst into developing various retail food products, such as the Good Catch plant-based seafood line, continuing to push the Wicked Healthy mission. Derek partnered with Tesco, the largest grocery chain in Britain, as head of plant-based innovation to bring Wicked Healthy to its grocery stores all across Europe, launching the Wicked Kitchen Foods line. Together, we've also launched a number of groundbreaking, plant-based foods and consulted with various restaurants and manufacturers. These new partnerships allow us to bring our love of plant-based cooking and eating to an even wider audience.

Yeah, we're plant pushers. At its core, though, Wicked Healthy is all about flavor. We spend most of our days in the kitchen developing and perfecting craveable, sexy food. That's how Derek came up with Ninja Squirrel sriracha, one of the top-selling, non-GMO hot sauces at Whole Foods Market. It's named after his backyard ninja squirrel, Zelda. (Yes, Derek trains squirrels.) If you want to taste something close to it, try our Homemade Badass Sriracha on page 276.

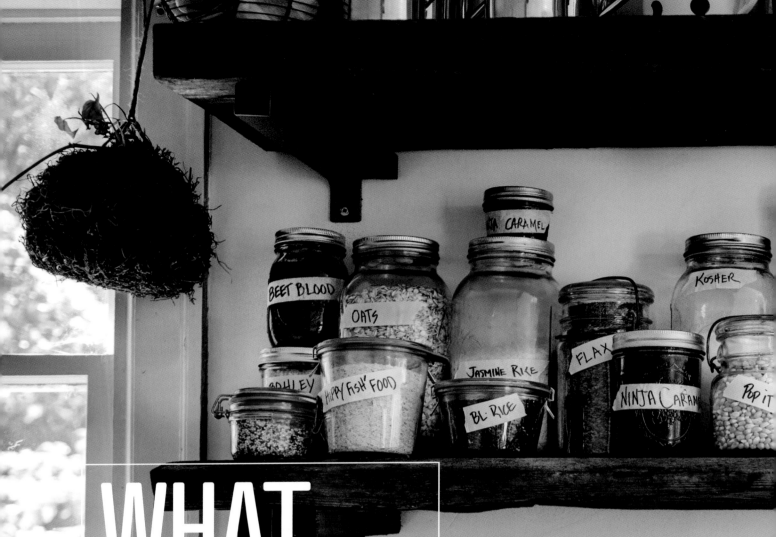

WHAT TO KEEP ON HAND

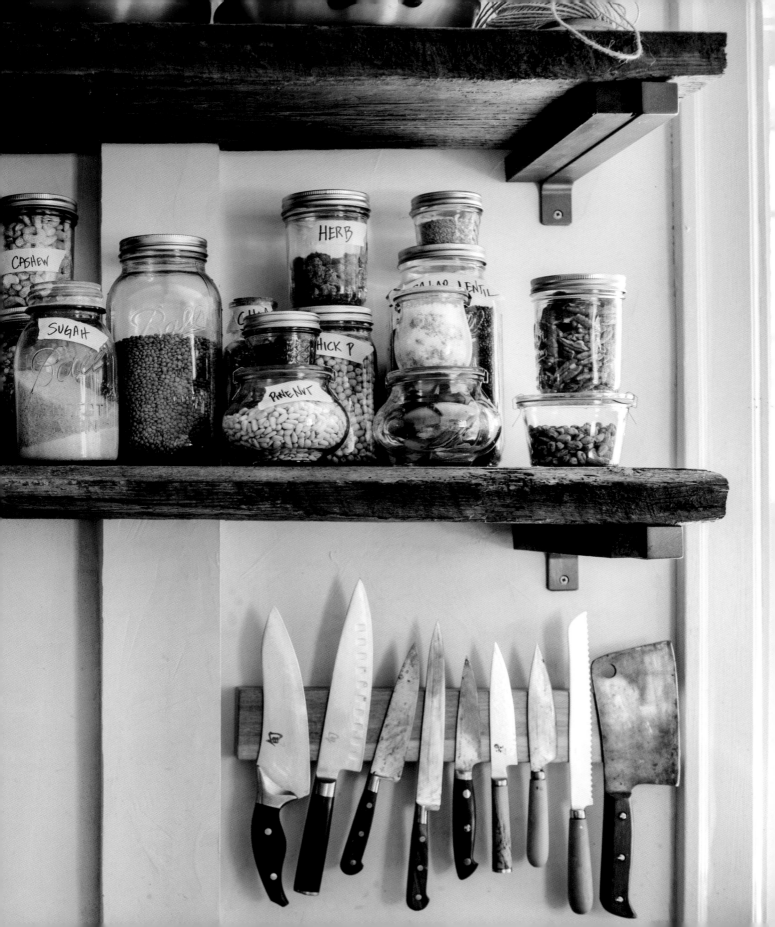

AN ORGANIZED COOK IS A SUCCESSFUL COOK. Here's the stuff we like to have in the kitchen. Don't worry. You don't have to go out and buy all these things—although, go for it, if you want! We included a few specialty items that we use only once in a while, like chocolate egg molds for the plant-based eggs in our Niçoise Salad (page 196). Most items, though, are everyday staples we use at every meal, like cutting boards and knives. For ingredients, we buy organic, local, and in season whenever possible, but you know, it's not always possible. If you're forced to choose between eating plant foods or not, buy whatever plant foods are available. The best news: Calorie for calorie, fresh plant foods almost always cost less than packaged processed foods. Why? Less packaging!

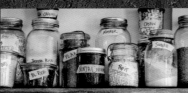
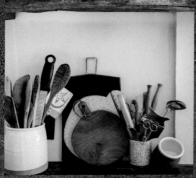

Equipment

PREP

WE LIKE STICK (IMMERSION) BLENDERS FOR SMALL AMOUNTS AND HOT SOUPS, TOO

Cutting board: a big one and a small one if you can—we like bamboo or Boos wood boards and season them with mineral oil every few months

Knives: chef's knife, serrated knife, and paring knife—skip the elaborate sets and spend your money on knives that feel balanced and comfortable to handle

Honing steel: inexpensive and keeps a knife's edge between professional sharpenings

Metal mixing bowls: small, medium, and large

Blender: high-speed blenders like Vitamix and Blendtec make silkier purees

Food processor: with various blades

Spice grinder: or coffee mill or mortar and pestle, for grinding whole spices and making pastes

MAKES MUSHROOM POWDER, TOO

Mandoline: essential for shaving vegetables wicked thin—handheld and countertop models are both great options—a truffle shaver also works

Microplane grater/ zester: for fine shreds of citrus peel, ginger, garlic, horseradish, nuts, and chocolate

A HEATPROOF EXTENSION OF YOUR FINGERS!

Tongs: short for the stovetop, long for the grill

Heat-resistant rubber spatulas: preferably small and large, to mix and scrape batters and such

Spider strainer: for fishing noodles and blanched vegetables from boiling water

Fine-mesh metal strainer: for straining purees

Salad spinner: a must—and this is your cue to eat more green salads

Plastic squeeze bottles: for storing sauces and making

dollops and dots on the plate

Tweezers: for a quick eyebrow adjustment

THESE ARE DIRT CHEAP AT RESTAURANT SUPPLY STORES

COOKING

Heavy-bottom sauté pans: 10-inch and 12-inch, for sautéing, searing, and pressing—cast-iron is wicked versatile; or use heavy clad metal pans with a stainless steel surface and copper or aluminum core

Cast-iron grill pan: if you don't have an outdoor grill—long rectangular grill pans that have a flat griddle on the other side do double duty

Wok: a 14-inch carbon-steel flat-bottom wok works great on gas and electric cooktops—keep it well seasoned and it's perfect for stir-frying, braising, poaching, and steaming (with bamboo steamers)—it also

doubles as an indoor smoker—and you can toss an entire pound of pasta with sauce in it!

Steam basket: a must for steaming, making dumplings, and reheating food

STACKABLE BAMBOO IS OUR FAVORITE—COOKS MULTIPLE FOODS AT THE SAME TIME

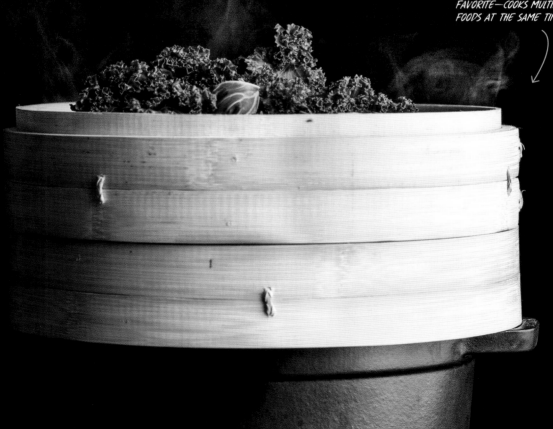

Pots: small, medium, and large saucepots for soups and sauces, plus one large stockpot (about 12-quart capacity) for boiling pasta and corn, making stocks, and making the occasional batch of stew for a crowd

Slow cooker: for fuss-free beans, chilis, soups, stews, and one-pot meals

Dutch oven: cast iron like Lodge or Le Creuset can go from stovetop searing to oven braising

 GREAT FOR BAKING FRESH BREAD, TOO

Baking dishes: at least a 2-quart (8-inch square) and 3-quart (13- x 9-inch pan) for brownies, gratins, casseroles, and such

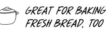 *A KETTLE-STYLE CHARCOAL GRILL CAN ALSO HANDLE EVERYTHING YOU THROW AT IT*

Baking sheets: several half-sheet pans for baking cookies, roasting vegetables, and holding food

Grill: for high heat, smoke, and cooking outside—we love to BBQ on the Big Green Egg

🖐 STORAGE

Clear jars: glass or plastic with tight-fitting lids for grains, beans, nuts, sprouting, etc.

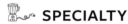 *SEEING FOOD IN CLEAR CONTAINERS INSPIRES US TO GET COOKING!*

Zipper-lock bags: gallons and quarts— where would we be without these!?

Commercial boxes of plastic wrap and aluminum foil: so much better and easier to use than what you can get in a grocery store—hit the restaurant supply store for these

🔌 SPECIALTY

Tortilla press: essential for Fresh Corn Tortillas (page 104)

VERY CHEAP!

Manual pasta roller: or KitchenAid attachment, for rolling out Pasta Dough (page 208)

Ice cream maker: or KitchenAid attachment, for Amaretto Gelato (page 230)

Silicone chocolate egg molds: for Plant-Based Eggs (page 198)—we use the 100 ml size from Silikomart

Dehydrator: for Plant Bacon (page 128), Nori Sunflower Snacks (page 55), and Olive Dirt (page 197)—Excalibur is our favorite or you could use a regular oven set to low convection

Juicer: for all kinds of healthy juice like Cucumber, Celery, Green Apple, and Kale Juice (page 248)— you could get by with a blender if you like pulp—we prefer the clear juice you get from masticating juicers like Omega

Ingredients

BEANS

Dried beans: Rancho Gordo is one of our favorite suppliers of heirloom dried beans

Canned beans: black, white, kidney, pinto, chickpeas

DID YOU KNOW THERE ARE MORE THAN 800 VARIETIES OF BEANS?!

Lentils: black, brown, French, red, split peas

QUICK-COOKING PROTEIN!

GRAINS, PASTAS, AND FLOURS

Rice: bamboo, basmati, black, brown, jasmine, white, wild

Whole grains: barley, bulgur, farro, kasha, millet, oatmeal (old-fashioned), popcorn, quinoa, steel-cut oats, wheatberries

DON'T FORGET—MOST WHOLE GRAINS HAVE 5–6 GRAMS PROTEIN PER SERVING

Flours: all-purpose flour, whole-wheat flour, chickpea flour, masa harina, tipo "00" flour, semolina, stoneground cornmeal

Dried pasta: choose your favorite shapes from elbows to penne to linguine—look for a rough surface on the pasta for the best quality and best texture to hold sauces

Starches: arrowroot, cornstarch, potato starch, tapioca—for thickening and breading

Bread crumbs: plain and panko

WHOLE-WHEAT PANKO IS GOOD—SO IS GLUTEN-FREE RICE PANKO

CONDIMENTS

Hot sauce: sriracha, sambal oelek or other fresh chile paste, local hot sauces, salsas

WE CHOOSE NINJA SQUIRREL FIRST!

Barbecue sauce: Austin's Own is a killer brand

Savory sauces: tamari (it's usually gluten-free) or soy sauce, miso paste

Creamy sauces: Plant-based mayo (Vegenaise and Just Mayo are our favorites—or make your own with the recipe on page 264), ranch dressing (Follow Your Heart rocks)

Pickles and mustards: kimchi, various pickles, a variety of mustards

Fruit jellies and jams: buy local or make your own with seasonal fruits

Stocks: Vegetable Stock (page 284) or store-bought stock (Massel, Better Than Bouillon, and NoBull are favorites), in case you run out of homemade

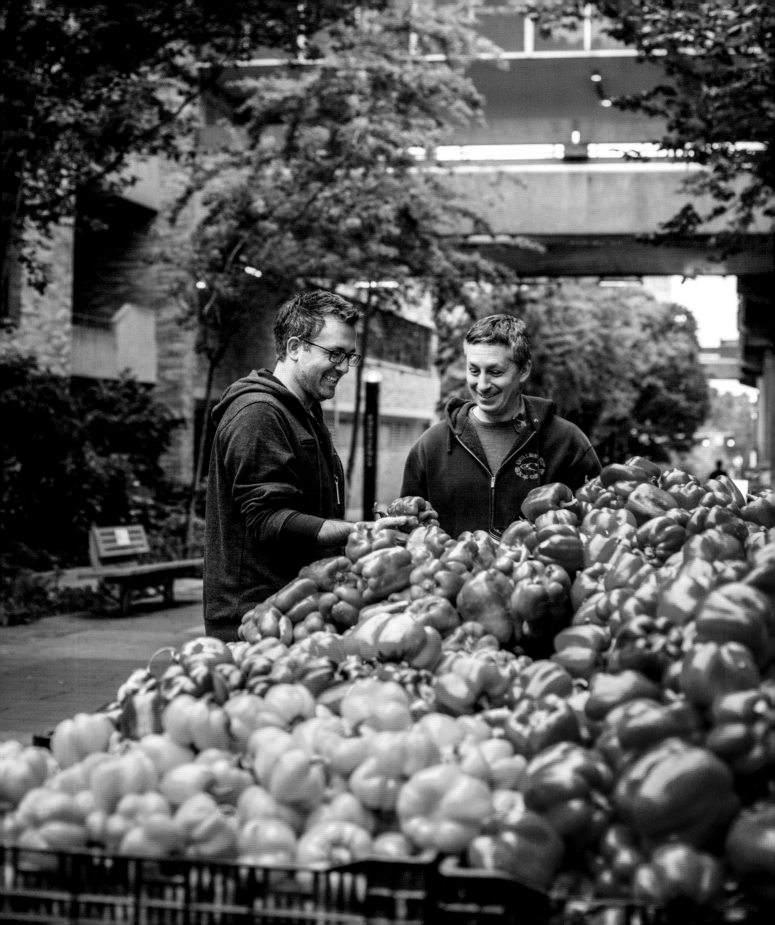

🥬 PANTRY VEGETABLES

Jars or cans: artichokes, capers, olives, tomato paste, plum tomatoes, diced tomatoes

🍇 DRIED FRUITS AND MUSHROOMS

Dried fruit: cherries, dates, currants, mangoes

GREAT FOR BUZZING INTO FRUIT POWDER

Freeze-dried fruit: pineapple, raspberries, strawberries, and other fruit (look for Karen's Naturals)

Dried 'shrooms: chanterelles, porcini, and shiitakes for flavoring sauces and stocks and for buzzing into mushroom powder for seasoning

🎃 NUTS, SEEDS, AND NUT BUTTERS

Nuts and seeds: almonds, cashews, hazelnuts, peanuts, pecans, pine nuts, pistachios, pumpkin seeds (pepitas), sesame seeds, sunflower seeds

BUY THESE RAW SO YOU CAN ROAST AND SEASON AS NEEDED

Butters: almond butter, cashew butter, natural peanut butter, tahini (sesame butter)

🥣 SEA GREENS

Dried seaweed: arame, dulse, kombu, nori, wakame, or other seaweeds for soups and bowls (toasted nori and crumbled dulse make good substitutes for finishing salt)

OILS, VINEGARS, AND COOKING WINES

Oils: everyday olive oil, vegetable oil, or grapeseed oil for sautéing; spray oil such as olive oil (Spectrum is a good brand—or refill a nonpump Evo sprayer with your favorite oil); good-quality extra-virgin olive oil for drizzling and fresh applications; specialty flavorful oils like walnut oil and toasted sesame oil for dressings, sauces, and drizzling

Vinegars and cooking wines: balsamic, black vinegar, cider vinegar, distilled vinegar, red wine vinegar, sherry vinegar, Pok Pok Som drinking vinegars, Marsala, Madeira, dry sherry, white and red cooking wines, Shaoxing wine

GREAT FOR STIR-FRY SAUCES AND IT'S CHEAP AS CHIPS

FIND THESE ONLINE—SOOOO GOOD IN SAUCES AND MARINADES!

🧂 SALT, SPICES, AND HERBS

Salt: fine and medium grain sea salt for general seasoning and baking (we like Portland's own Jacobsen), flake salt for finishing, smoked salts

Whole spices: Just a few—black peppercorns in a grinder, cumin, coriander, fennel seed, mustard seed, nutmeg, sesame seeds, vanilla beans (just slit and scrape out the vanilla seeds—much more flavor than extract)

*LASTS FOREVER—
GRATE AS NEEDED*

Ground spices: ancho chile, cardamom, cayenne pepper, chili powder, cinnamon, cloves, cumin, granulated onion and garlic, ginger, mustard powder, paprika and smoked paprika, poultry seasoning, red pepper flakes, white pepper for when you don't want

black pepper flecks in a white sauce or soup

Whole dried chiles: ancho, chipotle, pasilla, New Mexico

SO MANY MORE GREAT DRIED CHILES!

Dried herbs: bay leaves, oregano, rosemary, sage, thyme—to name a few

🍃 FRESH HERBS

Italian parsley, cilantro, mint, dill, chives, thyme, oregano, rosemary, sage (plant a small herb garden if you can—even on your windowsill)

YOU CANNOT HAVE ENOUGH FRESH HERBS

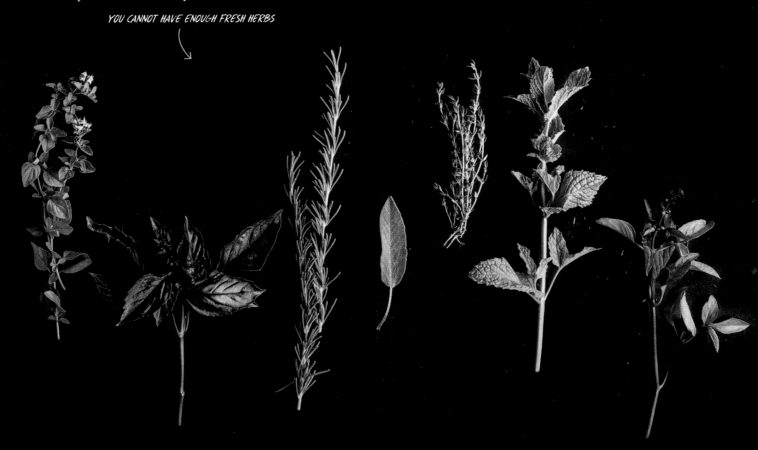

SWEETENERS

Granulated sugars:
coconut sugar,
turbinado sugar,
maple sugar, organic
cane sugar

Liquid sweeteners:
agave syrup, brown rice
syrup, maple syrup

Dried fruits: mango,
fig, date, apricot

BLEND INTO A PASTE WITH A LITTLE WATER FOR A WHOLE FOOD SWEETENER!

FRESH VEGETABLES AND FRUITS

Stock as many as you can eat and replenish your stash regularly

BUY LOCAL AND IN SEASON!

 ## NONDAIRY

Plant-based butter:
we like the taste of
Miyoko's Creamery
Butter or Earth
Balance sticks

PERFECT SLICES FOR SANDWICHES

Cheese: Chao and
Follow Your Heart
cheese, cream cheese
and ricotta (Kite Hill is
a fave), Parmesan (such
as Follow Your Heart),
mozzarella (Miyoko's
mozz is a good choice)

Milk: soy milk, almond
milk, coconut milk, or
other nondairy milk

Sour cream:
Follow Your Heart tops
the list again

Yogurt: we haven't
found one better than
Kite Hill

Miso: white, red, dark
(try South River—you'll
be happy you did)

FROZEN

Convenience foods:
burgers (beets make
Beyond Meat's Beyond
Burger look deliciously
red!); sausages (Field
Roast Italian and

chipotle are faves);
meatless crumbles; a
variety of fishless items
(look for Good Catch)

BEYOND MEAT IS GOOD

Frozen veg and fruit:
corn kernels, peas,
edamame, strawberries,
raspberries, peaches,
mangoes, blueberries

WHEN YOU CAN'T GET FRESH, USE FROZEN FRUIT FOR DRINKS, SMOOTHIES, AND SAUCES

BREAD

Whole-grain rustic loaf, corn tortillas, baguettes as needed

PREFERABLY FRESH— SEE PAGE 104!

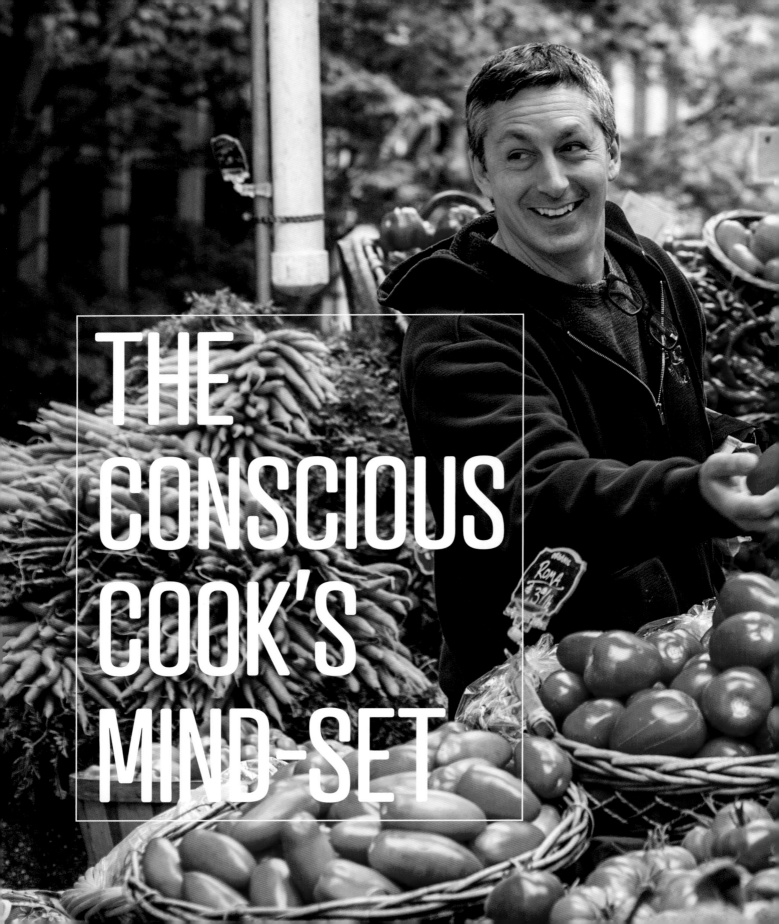

THE
CONSCIOUS
COOK'S
MIND-SET

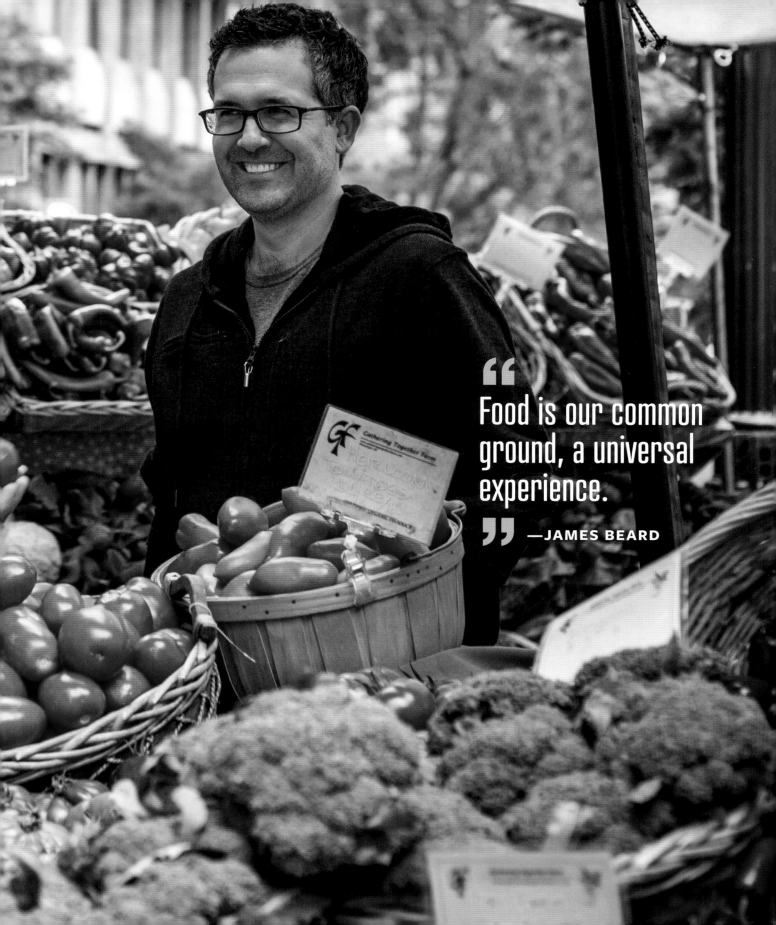

"
Food is our common ground, a universal experience.
"
—JAMES BEARD

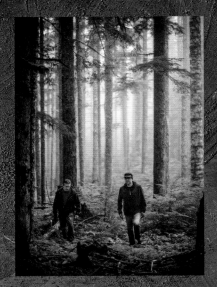

OUR NANA USED TO
SAY THE SAME THING!

SOME OF THE BEST CHEFS SAY THAT LOVE IS THE KEY INGREDIENT IN THEIR FOOD. It may sound a little out there, but there's something to it. Buddhists teach a similar concept called *tonglen*. It translates as "sending and receiving," and it's really about being compassionate, mindful, and present. It's useful for cooks because it reminds us that someone is on the other end of our food—the eating end. Let's keep them in mind as we're cooking. Food is an offering, and intentions should be clear. Ideally, you're cooking to feed people and nourish them, which is a big responsibility. It's great to surprise and delight them, too! Fundamentally, though, food is nourishment.

Food is powerful stuff—especially when you see its effects over time. It can hurt you and it can heal you. Just look at the top diet-related conditions out there—high blood pressure, heart disease, cancer, type 2 diabetes, osteoporosis. Scientists have studied them for years and have found that these conditions are definitely related to the foods we put in our bodies. The good news is that food can be potent enough to prevent these diseases and in some cases even help reverse these diseases. As one of the pioneers of the natural health movement, Ann Wigmore, put it, "The food you eat can either be the safest and most powerful form of medicine or the slowest form of poison."

Thankfully, there is one simple path to health: Eat more whole, minimally processed plant foods! It's common sense, right? Watch the movies *PlanEat*, *What the Health*, *PlantPure Nation*, *Forks Over Knives*, and *Food, Inc.*, and you'll see what we mean. If you eat heavily processed fast food all the time, it's going to affect you. You might gain weight. You might get depressed. But it will have some kind of health effect. Yes, fast food and junk food might taste good at first, but that's because they're engineered to satisfy your cravings for sugar, salt, and fat. Big food companies are in the business of selling lots of food. Period. They tend to be more focused on pushing your pleasure buttons than keeping you healthy.

The point is that being truly conscious as an eater, and as a cook, means recognizing that there's more to food than immediate gratification. Don't get us wrong—we love immediate gratification! But cooking puts the deeper power of food in your hands. With that power, you can heal people or hurt them. All we're asking is for you to see and hopefully use the power of food for good. Try to cook your own food instead of buying a lot of prepackaged crap. Even preparing a simple meal like Spaghetti with Nana's Red Sauce (page 202) gives you the ability to positively nourish yourself—and to nourish others. It can also provide emotional comfort food as you transition to healthier eating. That alone is a big epiphany for a lot of our clients and students. They start to see that cooking is so much more than getting dinner on the table. When you start bringing balance, nutrition, and awareness to your kitchen, it changes everything. You realize that you have the ability to positively affect yourself, your family, your friends, your health, and the health of the planet just by making dinner. One of the best places to take control of your future is at the end of your fork.

"WITH GREAT POWER COMES GREAT RESPONSIBILITY." —SPIDER-MAN'S UNCLE BEN (AND WINSTON CHURCHILL)

This realization is what gets many people into the kitchen in the first place. They cook to get a better handle on their own health. Everyone has their own preferences, and cooking lets you tailor what you eat to what you need or want. Want to cut back on salt? Use less salt and more spices! Want to avoid refined sugar? Use fresh and dried fruit instead! Too busy to cook from scratch? Use healthy convenience foods like canned tomatoes and canned beans! It doesn't matter whether you cook fancy or simple, or a little or a lot. It's just important to cook. Bottom line: Get your ass in the kitchen. It's the first and most important step toward taking control of your health. It's okay if you mess up now and then. Some of the greatest culinary discoveries are born from failures. Take a chance and step outside your comfort zone. You could be a total noob or a total pro in the kitchen. The fact is that no matter what skill level you're at, you will get better and better at cooking the more you do it.

TRY TO ADD SOME FRESH VEG AND GREENS TO WHATEVER PREPARED FOOD YOU BUY!

" Unless someone like you cares a whole awful lot, nothing is going to get better. It's not.

" —THEODORE SEUSS GEISEL (DR. SEUSS)

Get Organized

All professional chefs learn that an organized cook is a happy and sane cook. It's the first thing taught in culinary school. Just imagine going camping in the mountains. You want to make sure you have everything you need, so when you're out there, you don't suddenly find yourself up shit's creek without a paddle. A little planning and strategy actually save time and might mean the difference between eating highly processed junk and eating a nourishing home-cooked meal.

SET UP THREE PRIMARY AREAS. The main kitchen areas are for prep, cooking, and cleaning. Set up your prep area with maximum counter space.

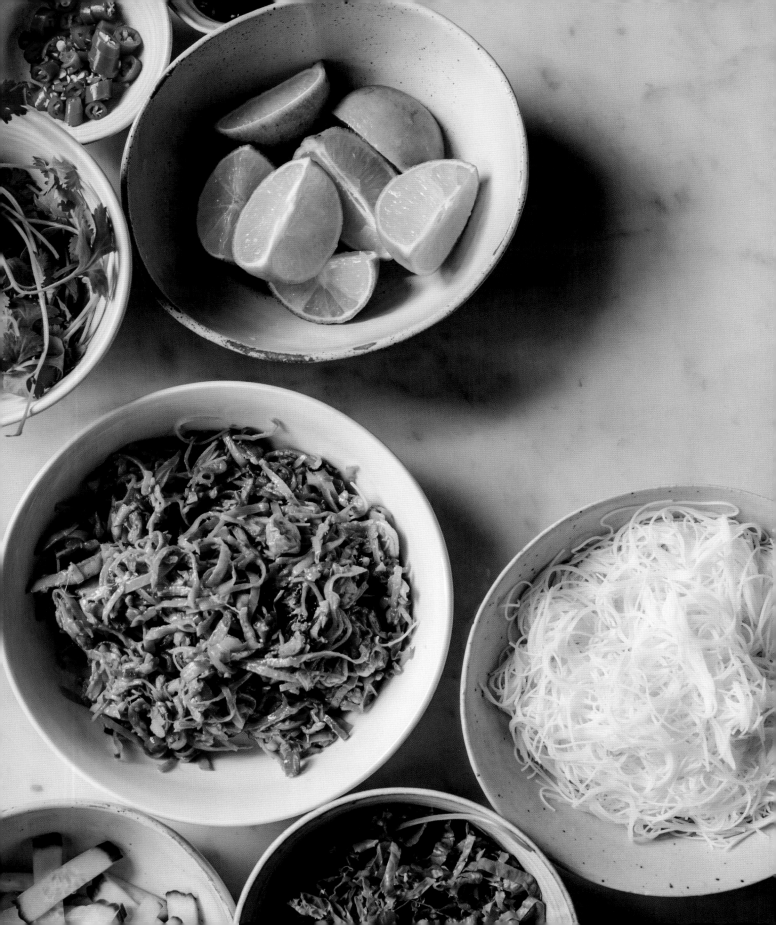

Appliances, mixing bowls, cutting boards, knives, and other prep equipment should all be nearby. It's helpful if basic ingredients like oil, salt, and spices are within reach. To free up counter space, think vertical. Can books or knives go on the wall? For your cooking area, store everything near the cooktop and oven—that's where you want all your pots, pans, wooden spoons, spatulas, tongs, and other cooking equipment. Ideally, the cooking area isn't too far from the prep zone so you're not running back and forth. For cleanup, think of the sink and dishwasher as anchors. Your cupboards and drawers should be nearby so you can quickly put away clean glasses, dishes, forks, spoons, and such. Derek uses the three-step rule. Everything you need should be within three steps of you while you're cooking.

RESET YOUR PANTRY FOR HEALTHY COOKING. Get rid of heavily processed foods, old spices and condiments, and anything you don't want to eat anymore. Out of sight, out of mind. Instead, fill your kitchen with whole, minimally processed foods. For snacks, look for dried fruits, nuts, and whole-grain crackers. Keep your pantry filled with whole grains like brown rice and farro, whole-grain flours, whole-grain pastas and breads, canned vegetables like tomatoes and artichokes, long-keeping vegetables like potatoes and winter squash, canned beans, dried beans and lentils, fruit spreads, jams, jellies, and a variety of hot sauces and salsas. Organize everything so it's easy to grab. Make a shelf for all the beans, another for the grains, another for the nuts and seeds. In your fridge and freezer, keep a steady supply of fresh seasonal vegetables and fruits; dark leafy greens; lettuces; fresh herbs; fresh juices; nondairy milk, yogurt, butter, and cheese alternatives (if these interest you); frozen fruits; and frozen vegetables like peas and corn kernels. When you step into an organized, well-stocked kitchen, the cooking goes so much faster, and it's so much more fun.

REPLACE DRIED HERBS ABOUT EVERY SIX MONTHS.

BATCH COOK. The idea of making a big meal on Sunday and then repurposing it throughout the week is a great one. It's all about stretching your meals. Roast whole heads of cauliflower or broccoli at a time. Roast a couple of batches of root vegetables like sweet potatoes, carrots, parsnips, onions, and celery root. Pan-sear or grill a slew of mushrooms. Make a big batch of Corona beans or lentils or a batch of rice or quinoa. We never cook beans or grains for just one meal. We always make a big batch. Maybe the beans are a side dish on Sunday, a taco filling on Tuesday, blended into a dip on Wednesday, and part of a soup on Thursday. Make a double recipe of Wicked Healthy Cheese Sauce (page 260), Nana Sarno's Red Sauce (page 265), or Mango Sriracha Caramel (page 270). You can freeze most sauces. Then just tweak them by adding different seasonings through the week. Batch cooking is the only way restaurants can turn out hundreds of meals a night. Avoid the dinnertime rush by doing the same thing at home.

THERE'S NO SUCH THING AS "LEFTOVERS." THEY'RE JUST COOKED INGREDIENTS WAITING TO BE TURNED INTO ANOTHER DISH!

READ THE RECIPE ALL THE WAY THROUGH.
Seriously, do this. Ever get halfway through a recipe and find you don't have an ingredient? Before you start cooking, give the recipe a quick read to avoid a mid-cook crisis. That also helps you strategize for efficiency. If both the taco filling and guacamole call for chopped onions, chop all your onions at once. Group similar tasks together, like getting all the ingredients from the fridge at one time, so you're not running back and forth. See page 49 for more on using our recipes.

MEEZ-ON-PLOSS

PRACTICE *MISE EN PLACE*. This French term literally means "put in place." Before you start cooking, get your equipment ready, prep your ingredients, and have everything you need measured out and ready to go. Getting prepped makes cooking so much faster, easier, and more fun. Stir-fry is a great example. The actual cooking

*MISE EN PLACE GOES WAY BEYOND THE KITCHEN. IT IS A STATE OF MIND.
—CHAD*

BASIC KNIFE TECHNIQUE

Don't be shy. Grab the knife like you mean it! Hold the handle but also the back edge of the knife right behind the heel of the blade. When your fingers hold some of the blade you get more control over the knife. Stand with the knife perpendicular to the food you're cutting. As you cut, keep the tip of the knife pointed down and let the blade and the weight of your body do most of the work. The knife should mostly move forward and backward to slice. It shouldn't take much downward force. With your other hand, hold the food. Arch your fingers like an eagle's claw to grasp the food, but tuck your thumb behind your fingers to keep from cutting yourself. It helps to rest the blade against your arched fingers. Then you can slowly move your arched hand and the knife blade together as you cut the food. Aim to cut food into same-size pieces so they cook at the same rate. There's also some research showing that different knife cuts, such as long slices on an angle, expose more surface area and release more flavorful compounds from the food. So try to cut the food the way it's suggested in the recipe. It makes a difference!

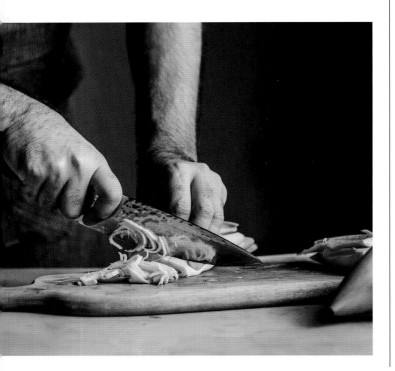

takes only a couple of minutes. Most of the work is chopping and mixing before you even heat up a pan. Get in the habit of prepping before you cook to make cooking less stressful. Mix your sauces, chop your vegetables, and marinate ingredients as far ahead of time as possible—even in the morning before you go to work.

MISE EN PLACE ALONE CAN SAVE YOU TONS OF KITCHEN STRESS!

CONSIDER TIMING. Look at what takes the longest and start those things first. Preheat the oven. Light the grill. Start the pasta water. Marinate the vegetables. Get those things going so you can prep other ingredients right before you start cooking. If you're organized and "mised out," you should have an idea of what to start cooking when and approximately when things will be done. Once you get faster with a knife, you'll be able to do some chopping while you've got pans on the stove.

WE LOVE CHOPPING—IT'S THERAPEUTIC!

HONE YOUR KNIFE SKILLS. We won't lie. Plant-based meals involve a lot of chopping. If you're short on knife skills, do some chopping in a food processor. Pick up a mandoline for quick slicing. Models that have julienne blades are even more useful, and they're pretty cheap these days. Even with fancy cutting tools, though, you will at some point be holding a chef's knife. Start with basic knife-holding technique to make chopping easier—and safer (see Basic Knife Technique at left). Keep those blades sharp! Every few uses, tune up your knife on a honing steel. Store your knives on a magnetic strip or in a knife block. Storing them loose in a drawer will only dull the blades.

REMEMBER: SHARP KNIVES CUT, DULL KNIVES SLIP!

COOK CLEAN. Even cats clean up their messes right away. Clean as you go! Get in the habit of discarding trash and wiping down countertops as you prep and cook. It's so much easier to get stuff done when the kitchen is clean. It calms your mind. Keep a clean towel folded near your workspace. Move food out of the way once it's prepped. Stack empty bowls and pans and move them to the cleanup area.

IF YOU EVER COOK WITH DEREK AND YOUR TOWEL IS LEFT UNFOLDED ON THE COUNTER, HE WILL FOLD IT FOR YOU. HE'S A BIT OCD ABOUT THAT. —CHAD

HAVE PATIENCE. Chopping and dicing get easier with practice. Cooking is a lot like riding a bike, yoga, and every other activity: The best way to get better at it is to do it more. It shouldn't be a drag and stressful—it should be fun! Just be patient and focus on your form. Speed will come. Your skills will develop. And then you'll be more confident and look forward to putting together meals that nourish your family, your friends, and yourself.

HALF OF BEING A GOOD COOK IS JUST SHOWING UP! —DEREK

> ### Pro Tip
> *To make dishwashing easier, soak dirty bowls and pans as soon as possible.*

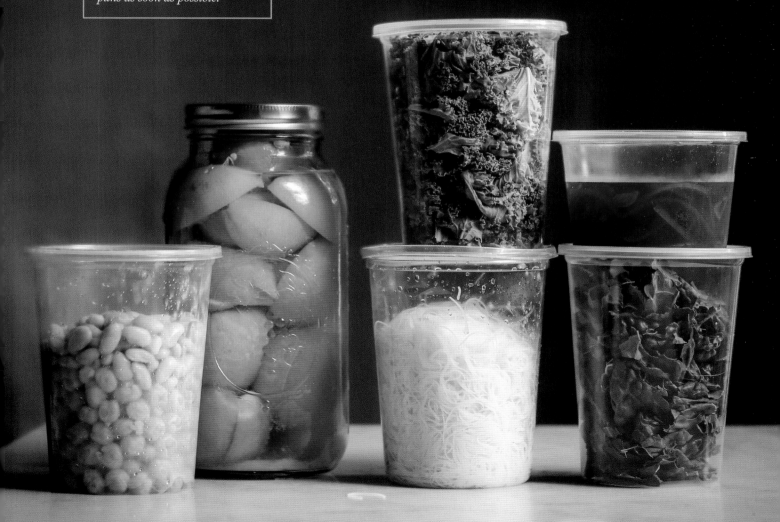

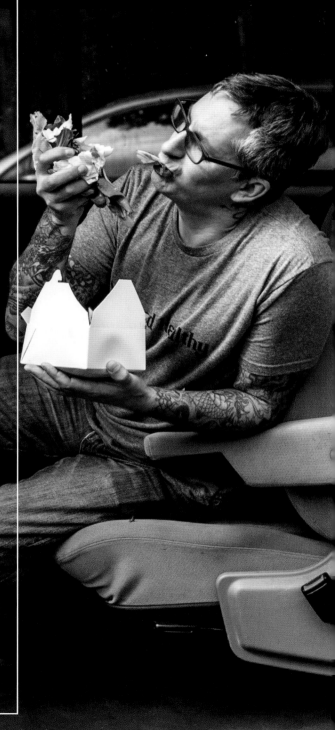

HEALTHY FOOD DOESN'T HAVE TO TASTE LIKE SHIT

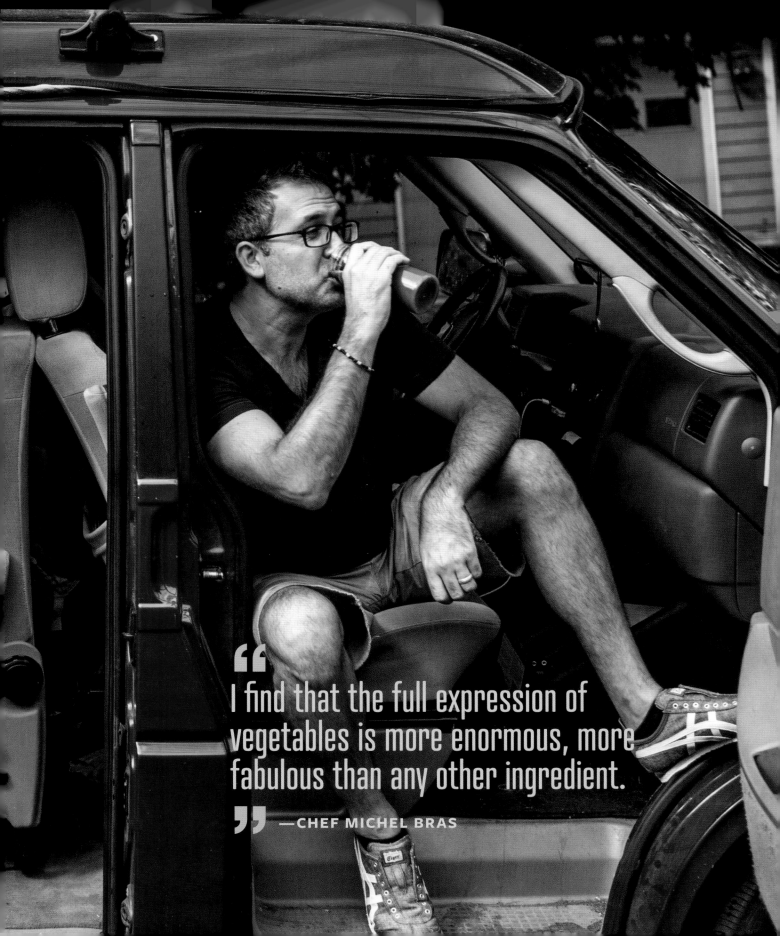

" I find that the full expression of vegetables is more enormous, more fabulous than any other ingredient. "
—CHEF MICHEL BRAS

SOME PEOPLE THINK THERE'S NOTHING GOOD TO EAT WHEN YOU'RE EATING HEALTHY. Are you kidding? Um...chocolate? Or how about avocados and strawberries; sandwiches, pasta, and tacos? When you stop to think about it, there's an amazing variety of awesome-tasting plant-based foods out there. We just need to eat more of them. In fact, one of the keys to a healthy diet, according to most doctors and nutritionists, is simply to eat a wide variety of plant foods.

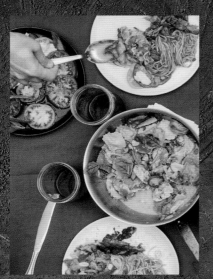

Choose the Best Ingredients

No matter what food you eat, there are two basic ways to put flavor on a plate:

1. Choose the best ingredients.
2. Use flavor-building techniques.

With ingredients, everyone has the same playing field—from professional chefs to home cooks. Choose the best-tasting food from the start and you're on your way to a great-tasting dish. When you can, buy local, seasonal, and organic. Shop your local farmers' market or healthy food store. Make sure the food is ripe, plump, and bursting with color and flavor. Of course, in a pinch, ingredients like frozen corn, peas, and butternut squash are fine, as are pre-cut vegetables like spiralized zucchini and pre-chopped carrots from the produce section of the store. Just keep in mind that flavor dissipates as soon as food is cut. For the absolute best flavor, buy whole foods and prepare them in your kitchen when your motivation is high. Practice your knife skills!

Go Easy on Adding Processed Sugar, Salt, and Fat

If you choose food wisely, your ingredients should taste good on their own without many—or any—enhancements. Then comes the real fun of combining ingredients and layering on the flavors. That's where creativity happens! Use a light hand with the sugar, salt, and fat. These three ingredients alone are linked to most of the health problems plaguing us today—from heart disease and high blood pressure to diabetes and obesity. It's *not* hard to see why. They taste great! In fact, we all need these ingredients in our bodies. Sugar provides calories for energy and is present in some form in nearly every food. Sodium is essential for keeping every cell in your body functioning properly. And fat keeps your nervous system running smoothly. Fat also helps you absorb fat-soluble vitamins like A, D, and E, and health-boosting nutrients like beta-carotene, lycopene, and lutein. We're kind of "hard-wired" to like the taste of sugar, salt, and fat. Food manufacturers know this simple fact. They tend to pile on the sugar, salt, and fat to make you crave their food products so you buy more.

We're not saying that all our recipes are sugar-free, salt-free, and fat-free. We use these ingredients—sometimes to wicked effect! The key thing to remember is that sugar, salt, and fat are highlight flavors in food—flavor enhancers, not substantial nourishment. When using sugar, salt, and fat in your cooking, think of them more like the special effects in a movie. You want a little sis-boom-bah here and there, but that's not the plot. Great-tasting beans, lentils, legumes, nuts, seeds, whole grains, vegetables, and fruits are the main story. Put those front and center.

If your taste buds have developed strong cravings for sugar, salt, and fat, then it's time to step back and start tasting real food again. Try a reset. Eat clean for a few days. Then buy a good-quality locally grown carrot in season, in the late spring or mid-fall. Eat it, unadorned. Taste it as you chew. You'll notice there's already quite a bit of sugar in a carrot. That is step 1 to understanding how to build flavors and how to season your food. Taste it!

Most foods already contain some sugar, salt, and fat—there's no need to automatically reach for those flavor enhancers. Taste as you go and try to save the sis-boom-bah for the end. The cook's process of seasoning and adding other ingredients is merely a matter of balancing the overall taste and texture of the foods you're working with.

Avocados are a good example. The average Hass avocado has 15% fat, 0.3% sugar, and 0.008% sodium. All that fat makes it taste rich and creamy. It's so low in sodium, however, that it tastes a bit bland. Maybe we sprinkle on a little salt at the end of prepping an avocado dish to balance the overall flavor. Or better yet, skip the salt, but add a whole-food source of sodium like olives or capers. Yum.

Tomatoes, another good example: The average tomato has only 0.2% fat and 0.005% sodium, with 3% sugar. If the tomato is ripe, it won't need any added sugar. It needs richness, though. Maybe you drizzle on a little olive oil and a pinch of salt to balance its natural flavors. Or, thinking back to the last example, avocados are a healthy source of fat, yet low in sugar. Maybe you combine the tomatoes with the avocados. Tomatoes bring sugar, avocados bring fat, and you could add in some olives and capers for sodium. Now you've got a tasty little salad going. No added sugar, salt, or fat needed!

Most chefs taste a dish multiple times so they know what seasonings to add along the way. That's cooking.

Hit All the Other Flavor Buttons

There's a lot of flavor to be had outside of sugar, salt, and fat. In fact, we perceive five basic tastes: sweet, sour, salty, bitter, and savory (or umami, as the Japanese call it). Notice that sugar and salt account for only two of those basic flavors. Sour is another basic taste that's wicked important. Sour flavors come in the form of acids in food, like the sharp tang of lemon juice and tart apples, or the puckery taste of sherry vinegar and red wine. Sour flavors are often overlooked in cooking. You should be adding them as a key element in most of your dishes. Adding a sour flavor can help a dish "pop" and balance all the other tastes in it—especially when you're cutting back on salt. Acidity can also be very subtle, like when you deglaze a pan with some wine and then simmer it off, leaving behind notes of acidity and sweetness.

Bitter is the tongue-tightening taste of bitter greens like arugula and broccoli rabe as well as certain beans like coffee and unsweetened chocolate.

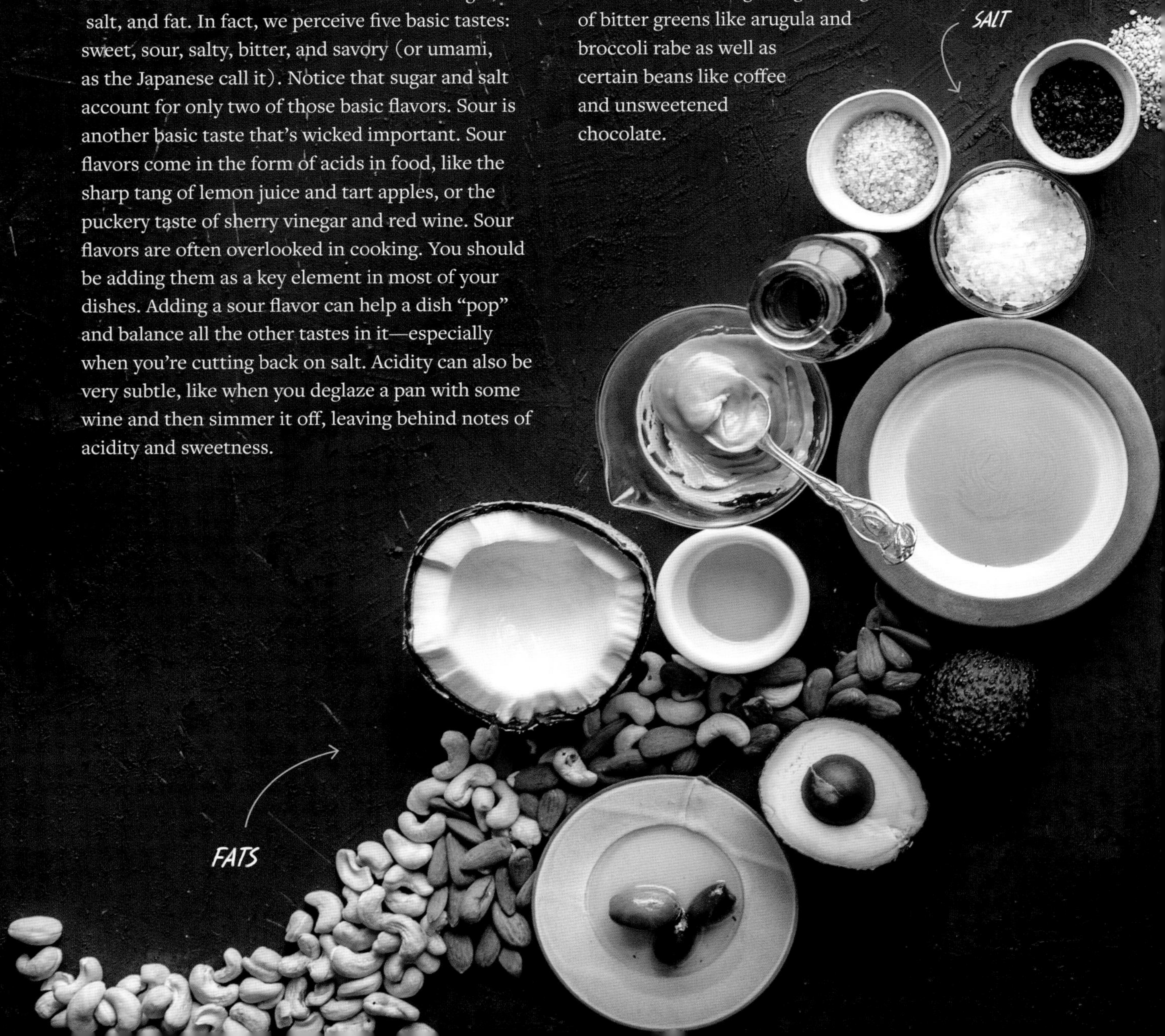

SALT

FATS

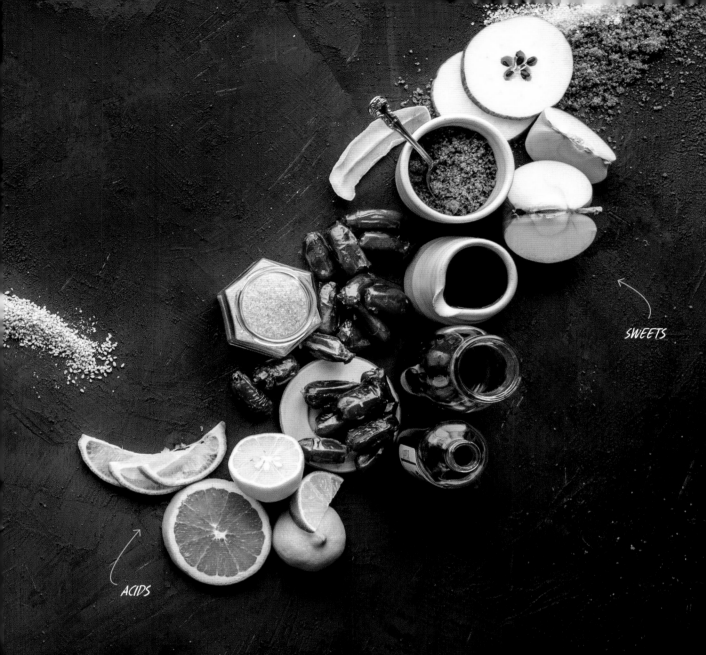

SWEETS

ACIDS

Bitterness will come naturally, and you'll probably be adding other ingredients to tame the bitterness—like adding soy sauce to bitter greens. Yes, salt (or in this case, soy sauce) tames bitterness. Fat can also dull the sharp taste of bitter foods.

The fifth taste, savory or umami, is the mouth-rounding flavor of things like mushrooms, potatoes, tomatoes, seaweed, and soy sauce. It's hard to describe: a little funky, a little earthy, and a lotta awesome. It gives you a total mouthgasm! (This is now a word.) This savory flavor is another basic, satisfying taste that helps to round out all the other flavors in a dish. Most vegetables have a savory element to them. If you need to immediately bump up the umami in a dish, add some mushrooms, mushroom powder, soy sauce, nutritional yeast, or seaweed like nori or dulse.

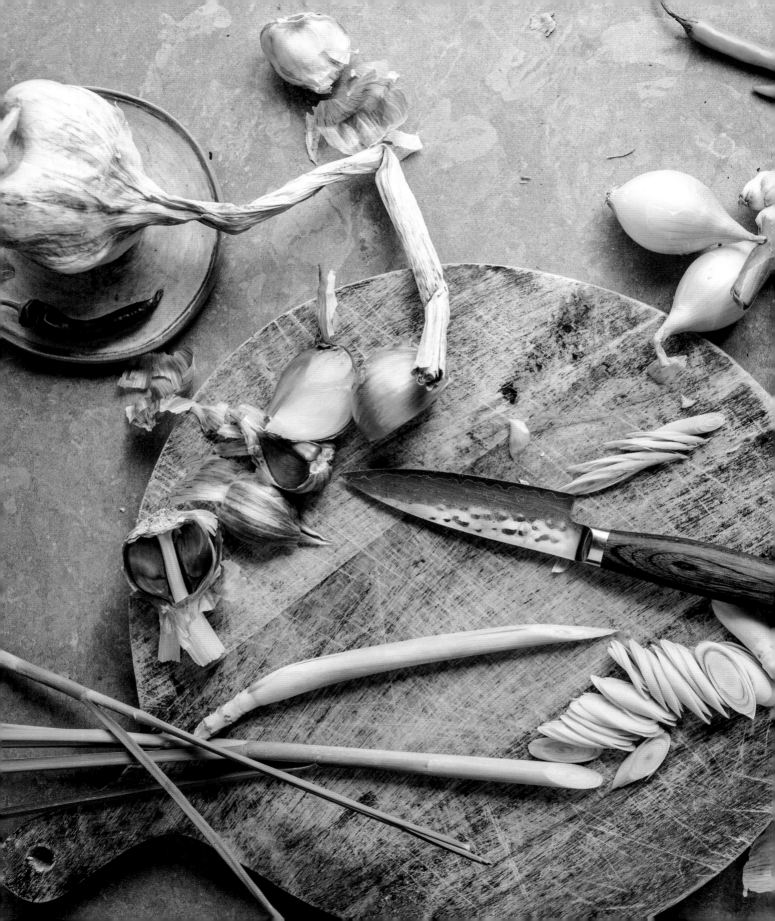

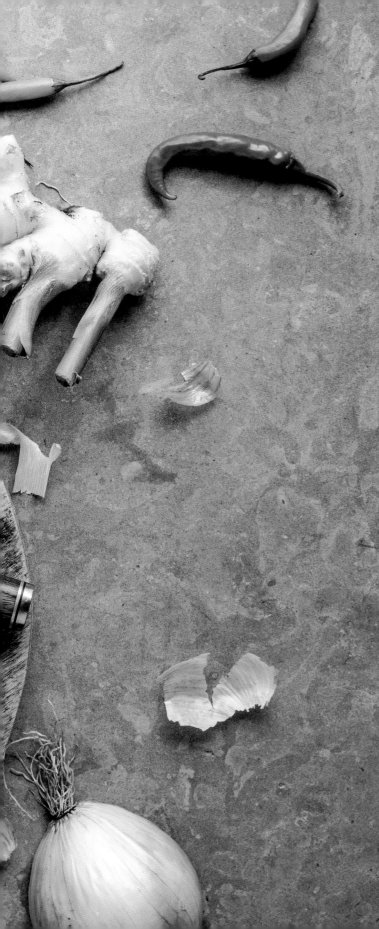

Add Layers of Flavor with Aromatics

Beyond the five basic tastes, there are dozens of other flavors in food. Consider the pungent taste of onions and garlic and the sharp taste of ginger and horseradish. We call these aromatics. They are often sautéed to start building flavor in a pan when you begin cooking a dish. Then there are the fresh green flavors of cilantro, basil, and other herbs, and the spicy flavors like those in chile peppers and black peppercorns. These three categories of flavor—aromatics, herbs, and spices—are absolutely critical to making healthy food taste its best. Plus, aromatics, herbs, and spices are healthy in and of themselves!

Think of the sugar, salt, and fat in food like the tripod of a stool: the basics. Once you've balanced those out by combining ingredients or adding seasoning, you round out the whole flavor profile with some sour, bitter, and/or savory tastes. From there, you layer on even more flavor with aromatics, herbs, and spices. That's how you make something like plain old chickpeas taste amazing—even if you don't cook anything but the chickpeas themselves. Need proof? Mix some cooked chickpeas with something sweet like chopped fresh tomatoes, something sour like fresh lemon juice, a little fat like olive oil, some aromatics like chopped onions and garlic, some chopped fresh herbs like basil and parsley, and some spices like red pepper flakes. Boom! Now you have a delicious dish of Italian-style chickpeas. Swap in some fresh mint instead of the basil and some ground cinnamon instead of red pepper flakes, and you have something closer to a Middle Eastern–style dish of chickpeas! Every cuisine in the world has its own signature flavors. But they're all built on the basic tastes of sweet, sour, salty, bitter, and umami, augmented with different aromatics, herbs, and spices.

Pay Attention to Aroma

The vestibule of the late Charlie Trotter's restaurant in Chicago always smelled incredible. Chef Charlie Trotter said that he had a vent installed from his baking ovens so that the aromas of fresh bread and pastries would flow directly into the vestibule. In the fall, you'd also get a whiff of caramelized apples and cinnamon. Then you'd walk into the restaurant and see a display of red, pink, and green apples and bright fall leaves in brick red, fire orange, and lemon yellow colors. By the time you sat down, your senses were on fire—and that's before you had anything to eat! The truth is, eating is far more than taste. It stimulates all the senses, particularly our sense of smell. Aroma is closely associated with our most powerful food memories, and, according to food scientists, most of what we call flavor is actually perceived as aroma.

When combining ingredients to put together a dish of food, think to yourself, "How is this dish going to smell? What can I do to engage the nose?" Aromatics, herbs, and spices come to mind right away—and for good reason. They smell great! Need flavor in a dish? Add herbs and spices. Always keep a wide variety of fresh and dried herbs and whole and ground spices in your kitchen (see page 18 for a list). Yes, fresh herbs are perishable, so grow a little kitchen windowsill herb garden if you can. Or at least keep one or two fresh herbs in your fridge at all times—like parsley and cilantro. They're pretty cheap and easy to replenish. Adding that burst of freshness can make a world of difference in a dish.

Add delicate fresh herbs like parsley, cilantro, and basil near the end of cooking. These herbs lose flavor if you add them too early. We also prefer not to puree fresh herbs—unless we're making an herb sauce like pesto, chutney, or herb oil. The reason: Delicate fresh herbs are like an upper stair on the foundations of flavor created by the aromatics and the beans, lentils, legumes, grains, vegetables, or fruit you are preparing. If you puree the fresh herbs, their flavor sinks into the foundation and you lose that layer of taste. Think of all your ingredients as layers of flavor that you build from the bottom up. Keep the layers.

Sturdier herbs like rosemary, thyme, and bay leaves can be added a little earlier in the cooking process because they need more heat to release their aromas. When we make a pot of beans, for instance, we add whole sprigs of rosemary or thyme at the beginning of cooking. As the beans simmer, the herb leaves naturally fall off the stems, and you can just remove the stems before serving the dish. Of course, you could just mince these hearty herbs to release their flavor, and add them a little later in the cooking process. It's up to you. Both heat and chopping release the aromas inside herbs.

As for spices, we use them whole and ground—and lots of them. We like bold-flavored food. Black peppercorns are always in a grinder at the ready. We also keep plenty of spices like granulated onion and garlic, ground ginger and turmeric, and a variety of ground chili powders (from cayenne to smoked paprika) on hand. We love spicy food so much that we usually have some fresh chiles in our kitchen, too—from skinny red Thai chiles to plump, spicy-sweet Fresnos. *MY FAVORITE! —DEREK*

DON'T BE BASHFUL WHEN USING THESE! —DEREK

Spices and herbs are critical components in all cooking—especially healthy cooking. As you're preparing a dish of food, take a whiff now and then. If it smells good, it will taste good. If the food doesn't smell robust enough to you, add some spices, herbs, and/or aromatics to bump up the aroma. Or use some flavor-building techniques.

HOW TO USE OUR RECIPES

Before you start cooking, read the recipe all the way through, including the Pro Tips and Options. You don't want to miss anything important, like substitutions you could use if you don't have a particular ingredient or flavor variations that you might prefer. You'll notice that some recipe components appear as stand-alone recipes. This is one of the key teachings in this book: If you break the work of cooking into small, manageable chunks, a complex dish doesn't seem like such a chore. It also gets you in the habit of keeping some flavor bombs in your fridge and pantry. And that makes cooking on the fly so much faster and easier!

Salt: We call for sea salt in most recipes. It's usually medium-fine in texture, but we also use fine sea salt for baking and flaky sea salt for crusting and sprinkling here and there. Look for sea salt that's roughly equivalent in size to Diamond Crystal kosher salt. That means every teaspoon of salt should weigh about 3 grams.

IF YOU WANNA GET TECHNICAL!

Sugar: For granulated sugar, we like vegan organic cane sugar because it's not filtered through charred animal bones like white sugar. The same goes for turbinado (raw), demerara, muscovado, and coconut sugars, which we use instead of plain ol' brown sugar.

Oil: We use mild-tasting oil for most sautéing, roasting, dressings, etc. Everyday olive oil, vegetable oil, and grapeseed oil are favorites. Occasionally, we use specialty oil for flavor—mostly that means good-quality extra-virgin olive oil, toasted sesame oil, walnut oil, pumpkin seed oil, or another nut or seed oil.

Measurements: We sometimes list *½ tablespoon* in our recipes. No, sets of measuring spoons don't normally include a ½-tablespoon measure. Just fill the 1 tablespoon measure halfway. If you want to be more precise, ½ tablespoon = 1½ teaspoons.

Vegetables: We call for whole vegetables whenever possible to make shopping easier. Sometimes we call for large or small vegetables, such as onions. If the size is not specified, use a medium one.

Remember: A recipe is like a road map. It's useful, but to get where you're going, you still have to drive the car. That means you're still the one doing the cooking. That's what makes it exciting. You're in control! You can make whatever you want! Just keep in mind that ingredients change, ovens have hot spots, and your pan may be thick or thin or conduct heat quickly or slowly. Pay attention while you're cooking. The recipe isn't gospel. It's a guide. Smell the food, taste it, and take the wheel. You're in the driver's seat. Look at the food not at the clock. The food will tell you when it's browned enough or ready to eat.

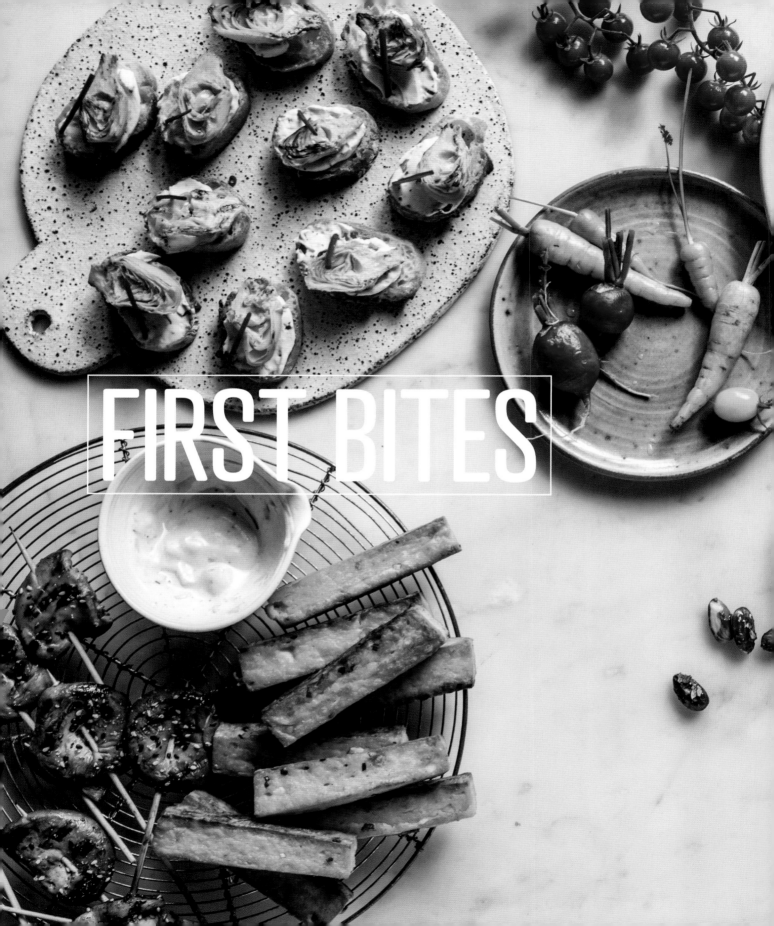

FIRST BITES

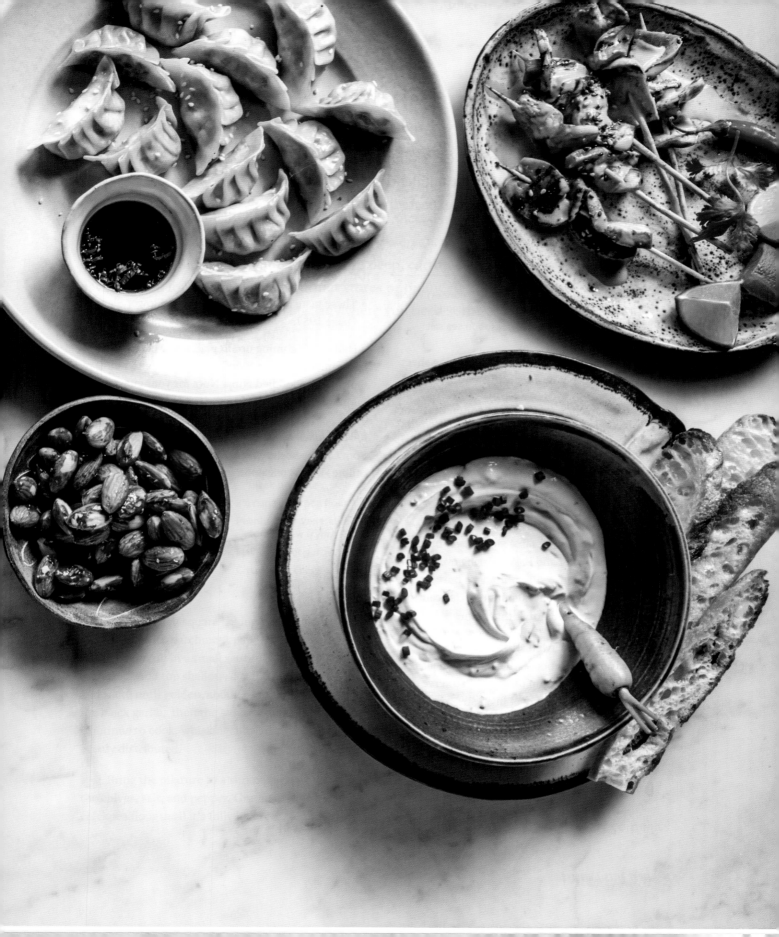

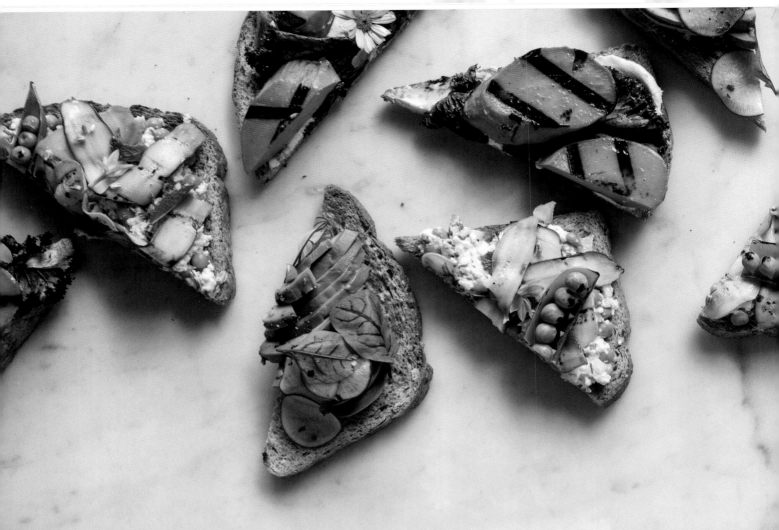

AVOCADO TOASTS *with*
RADISHES *and* MEYER LEMON

I love kicking off the day with this snack. It hits all the right texture and flavor buttons—crunchy, creamy, spicy, juicy, salty, tart, earthy, rich...what a way to wake up! I pick fresh radishes from the garden and shave a few slices over each toast. If you can find it, add some crunchy spirulina. I use Sunfood spirulina from Costa Rica—the perfect superfood addition. Sometimes I also replace the salt with a dusting of Olive Dirt (page 197). —*CHAD*

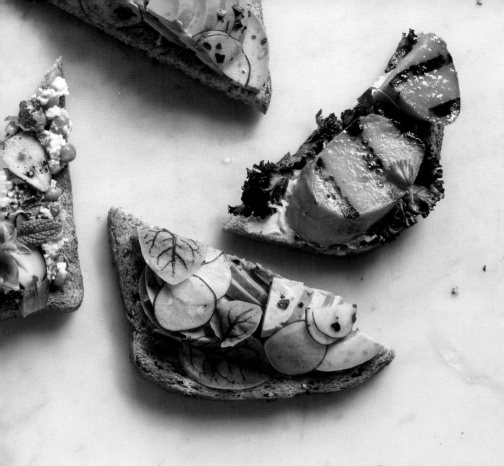

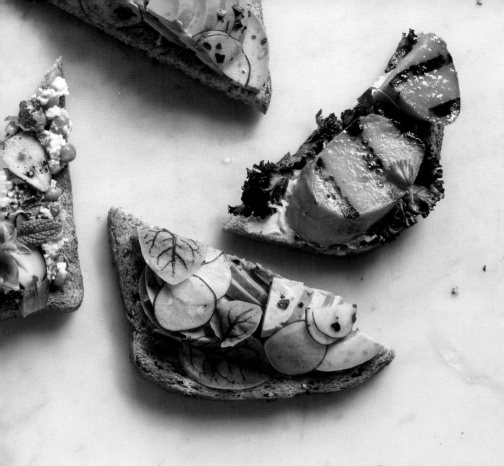

![toast icon] **SERVES 2**

---

4 big slices whole-grain
    seeded bread

1 ripe avocado, pitted and
    peeled

3 or 4 small Easter egg or
    breakfast radishes

2 tablespoons coarse
    spirulina, optional

Pinch of flake salt,
    such as Maldon

Pinch of red chile flakes

Freshly cracked black
    pepper

Handful of baby greens,
    such as sorrel

1 Meyer lemon, halved

1 Lightly toast the bread, then spread one-fourth of the avocado over each slice.

2 Use a mandoline or truffle shaver to slice the radishes paper-thin and then arrange in an even layer over the avocado.

3 Sprinkle each toast with spirulina (if using), flake salt, chile flakes, and black pepper. Top with baby greens, and squeeze a little Meyer lemon juice over each toast before serving.

MINTED PEA RICOTTA, GRILLED ZUCCHINI, *and* CHARRED LEMON TOASTS

Serve this fresh green toast for brunch in the spring. Or try it anytime as a snack. Be sure to shave the zucchini into super-thin ribbons. I like to mark them briefly on a grill for more flavor and sexiness. They lend the toast height, color, and crunch. —*CHAD*

 SERVES 2

½ small yellow summer squash

½ small green zucchini

Spray or drizzle of olive oil

1 lemon

4 slices seeded whole-grain bread

1 cup Minted Pea Ricotta (page 64)

Garlic or chive flowers, optional

Small handful of mint leaves

Flake salt, such as Maldon

Freshly cracked black pepper

1 Heat a grill or grill pan to medium high. Use a mandoline or truffle shaver to slice the squash and zucchini into wicked-thin ribbons. Lightly drizzle or spray each ribbon with olive oil, then grill briefly to mark both sides.

2 Cut the lemon in half and grill cut-side down until lightly charred, 2 to 3 minutes. Grill each slice of bread until lightly toasted but not burnt, a few seconds per side.

3 Spread ricotta on each slice of toast and top with the sliced grilled zucchini and squash, overlapping and twisting a couple of slices for a better aesthetic. Sprinkle on the garlic flowers (if using), a few leaves of mint, a flick of flaked sea salt, and some cracked black pepper.

4 Just before serving, squeeze the charred lemon over the toast.

OPTION

- Garnish the toasts with English peas (in the shells).

GRILLED BABY ARTICHOKE CROSTINI
with CASHEW CRÈME FRAÎCHE *and* HORSERADISH

At dinner parties, I usually start us off with crostini as one of the small bites. The crunchy, creamy combo sets the right tone. This one is especially good with fresh baby artichokes. Just trim down fresh baby chokes to the tender yellow-white hearts, steam, and cut in half. Then give them a good pan-sear to develop some flavor. Too busy for all that? You can sear pre-trimmed jarred or frozen baby artichoke hearts instead. But steer clear of quartered marinated artichoke hearts in olive oil and vinegar: Those won't work here. Either way, the real star is fresh grated horseradish. It adds the perfect zing! —*CHAD*

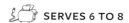 **SERVES 6 TO 8**

1 small baguette, about 8 ounces

2 tablespoons everyday olive oil, plus a little for pan-searing

Coarse sea salt and freshly ground black pepper

½ cup plain plant-based cream cheese, such as from Kite Hill

¼ cup Cashew Sour Cream (page 77) or Plant-Based Mayo (page 264)

2½ tablespoons freshly zested horseradish or 1½ tablespoons prepared, plus some for garnish

2 tablespoons minced fresh chives, plus a few ½-inch pieces for garnish

2 teaspoons grated lemon zest

1 cup whole baby artichoke hearts, drained (or thawed if frozen)

1 For the crostini, preheat the oven to 375ºF.

2 Slice the baguette into thin (⅛-inch) slices (no more than ¼ inch thick). Drizzle or brush the slices all over with the olive oil and sprinkle with salt and pepper. Arrange the slices in single layers on baking sheets and bake until crisp and golden, 5 to 7 minutes. Remove from the oven and set aside.

3 In a small bowl, mix the cream cheese, sour cream, horseradish, chives, and lemon zest. Taste, then season with salt and black pepper until it tastes good to you. Mix thoroughly and use immediately or refrigerate for up to 3 days. (An easy way to store and use this is to spoon it into a pastry bag or zipper-lock bag; then you can just pipe it onto the crostini.)

4 Halve the artichokes lengthwise and season lightly with salt and pepper.

5 Heat a heavy pan such as cast iron over medium-high heat. When hot, drizzle or spray in a little oil, then carefully place the artichokes cut-side down in the pan. Pan-sear until golden brown, about 3 minutes.

6 To assemble, spoon a dollop of the cream cheese mixture on each crostini, then top with an artichoke half. Garnish with freshly zested horseradish and some chive pieces.

FIERY BLACK BEAN SPREAD

Slather it on corn bread. Add it to your Taco Bar (page 112).
Or serve it with sliced jicama for dipping.

 MAKES ABOUT 2 CUPS

---

1 white onion, chopped

3 tablespoons everyday
  olive oil

2 cups cooked or rinsed
  canned black beans

3 tablespoons sriracha

Pinch of sea salt

1 In a medium skillet, sauté the onion in
1 tablespoon of the oil over medium heat until
golden brown, 6 to 7 minutes.

2 Transfer to a food processor along with the
remaining 2 tablespoons olive oil and everything
else. Blend until not quite smooth; it's nice to keep
it a little chunky. This dip keeps refrigerated for
up to 5 days.

5 Soak a handful of wooden skewers in water to cover for 30 minutes. When ready to cook, preheat the oven to 350°F. Thread each strip of mushroom on a skewer, making as many ribbon folds as possible without breaking the mushroom. Place the skewers on a baking sheet and bake in the hot oven until lightly browned, 20 to 30 minutes.

6 *FOR THE SAUCE*: Combine all the ingredients in a blender and buzz it all up until smooth. For a thicker sauce, use less water; use more to make it thinner.

7 Drizzle a little sauce over the skewers before serving with the remainder on the side for dipping.

OPTIONS

- Switch it up and use almond butter or cashew butter in the sauce instead of peanut butter.

- Garnish with fresh cilantro, chopped chiles, and lemon or lime wedges for squeezing.

> **Pro Tip**
> *Use the leftover mushroom caps to make Mushroom Stock (page 284) or add them to the filling for Porcini Ravioli (page 211). Or just sauté them, toss with tamari, and add to your favorite noodle bowl.*

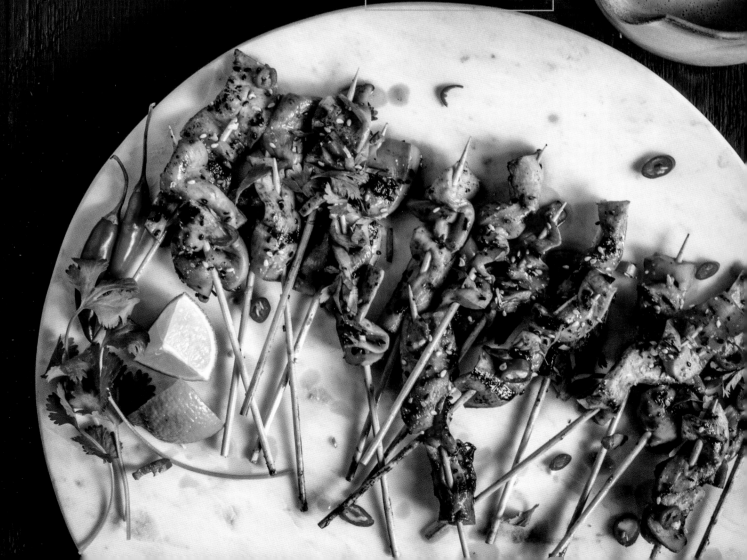

SMOKY POUTINE

If we had a restaurant, this hearty, messy, filling dish would be on the bar menu. The name *poutine* alone makes us want to stick our faces in a plate of cheese fries with mushroom gravy. A little smoked paprika in the mix makes our heads swirl. Wash down the fries with a crisp pilsner or, if you're into that sort of thing, a hipster AF local IPA.

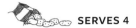 **SERVES 4**

4 russet potatoes, scrubbed

2 tablespoons mild-tasting oil

1 cup Mushroom Gravy Train (page 263)

1 cup Wicked Healthy Cheese Sauce (page 260)

½ cup (4 ounces) chive or plain plant-based cream cheese, such as from Kite Hill

½ teaspoon flake salt, such as Jacobsen's

¼ teaspoon smoked paprika

1 Preheat the oven to 425°F.

2 Cut the spuds lengthwise into wedges about ¼ inch thick. Leave the peels on so they get nice and crispy in the oven. Toss the wedges onto a baking sheet and rub all over with a little oil. Roast until the potatoes are soft in the middle and crispy brown all over, 30 to 40 minutes.

3 Meanwhile, warm up the sauces. Serve the spuds on a platter drizzled with the gravy and sauce and dolloped with plenty of cream cheese. Mix together the salt and paprika and flick it over the poutine.

> **Pro Tip**
> *If you want this dish ready to rock at a moment's notice, make the gravy and sauce up to a day or two ahead and pre-bake the potatoes at 350°F until tender inside, 30 minutes or so. Let them cool on the baking sheet, then chill in the fridge. When it's snack time, bake the spuds as directed until browned (it should take only 15 to 20 minutes since they're pre-cooked). Heat up the gravy and sauce and put it all together.*

OPTION

• To get more wicked, top the poutine with sliced red chiles, cilantro leaves, and green onions.

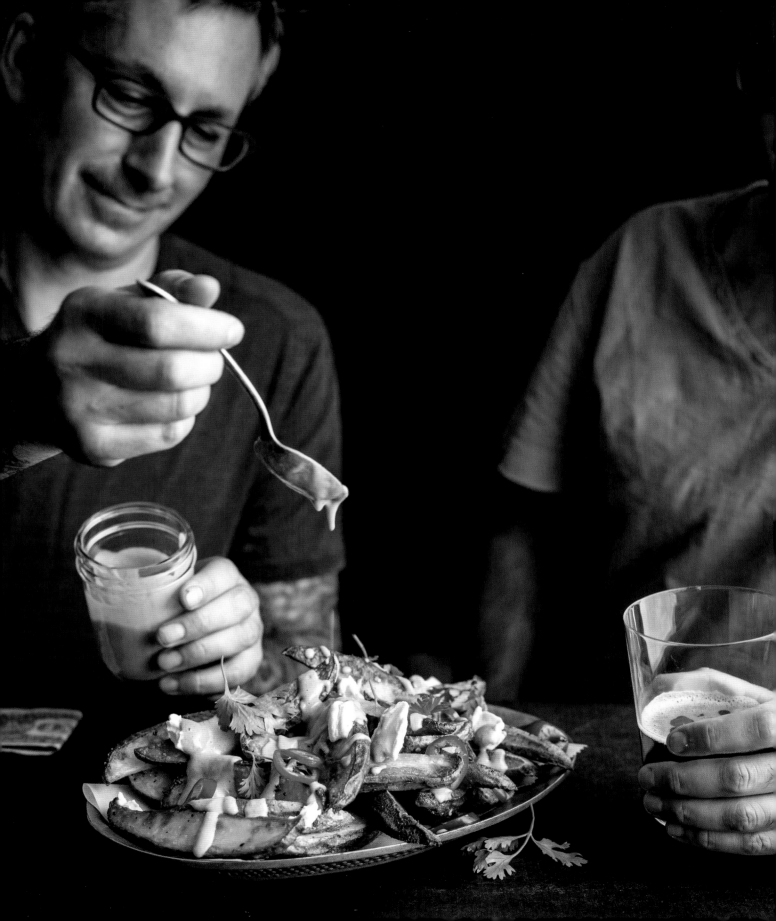

CASHEW AU POIVRE TORTE
with BASIL PARSLEY PESTO

When I was a staff chef at Living Light Culinary Institute, the founder, Cherie Soria, was the first to school me on making nut-based cultured cheeses. This "torte" is a takeoff on that idea, with layers of cashew cheese and basil pesto, a crust of pink peppercorns and chives, and a drizzle of sweet-tart syrup made from reduced (boiled down) white balsamic vinegar. The torte is about the size and shape of a small wheel of Brie cheese, and you serve it the same way...with crackers or bread as part of a plant-based cheese platter or to accompany a vegetable carpaccio board. The cashew cheese here is basically plant-based cream cheese—you can use it as a creamy base for almost anything. —*CHAD*

 SERVES 4 TO 6

CASHEW CHEESE

2 cups raw cashews

½ cup lukewarm filtered water

¾ teaspoon potent probiotics powder, preferably from New Chapter

1½ teaspoons onion powder

½ tablespoon sea salt

¼ teaspoon ground white pepper

¼ teaspoon fresh grated nutmeg

ASSEMBLY

3 tablespoons crushed pink peppercorns

3 tablespoons minced fresh chives

½ tablespoon flake salt

½ cup Basil Parsley Pesto (page 75)

½ cup white balsamic vinegar

1 FOR THE CASHEW CHEESE: Soak the cashews overnight in tap water to cover at room temperature.

2 Put the lukewarm filtered water in a blender (preferably high-speed). Add the probiotics powder and let stand a minute or two until dissolved.

3 Drain the cashews and transfer to the blender. Blend on medium to medium-high speed until very smooth, stopping to scrape and stir as necessary. Use a rubber spatula to scrape the mixture into a glass or ceramic bowl. Cover with a clean kitchen towel and let stand at room temperature until cultured, 14 to 16 hours. At this point, the probiotics will have grown, coagulated the protein in the mixture, and firmed up the cheese a bit.

4 The next day, when finished culturing, use the rubber spatula to stir the onion powder, salt, pepper, and nutmeg into the cheese.

5 TO ASSEMBLE THE TORTE: Grab a small springform pan or small round mold 4 to 5 inches in diameter and line with plastic wrap. Or find a mini-terrine mold or very small baking dish (2- to 3-cup capacity) and line with plastic wrap. Sprinkle the pan bottom with the peppercorns, chives, and salt.

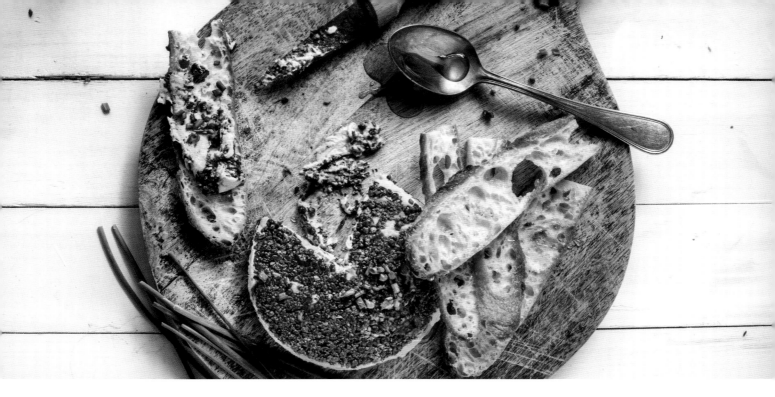

6 Press half of the cashew cheese firmly into the pan. Spread all the pesto in a thick layer over the cheese. Spread on the remaining cashew cheese. Cover and chill until firm, 1 to 2 hours.

7 Boil the vinegar in a small saucepan over high heat for about 10 minutes, until reduced in volume by about half, about ¼ cup. Let cool in the pan, up to 2 hours if you like.

8 Invert the torte onto a small plate and remove the pan and plastic wrap. Drizzle with the white balsamic syrup.

Pro Tip

Don't have time to culture? Omit the probiotics and replace with 2 tablespoons lemon juice. The end result will be slightly different but still a similar flavor profile, just without the zing.

BASIL PARSLEY PESTO

 MAKES ABOUT ½ CUP

2½ cups fresh basil leaves

¼ cup fresh parsley leaves

½ cup pine nuts

2 small cloves garlic, peeled

¾ teaspoon sea salt

A few grindings of black pepper

¼ cup everyday olive oil

Put everything but the oil into a food processor and pulse until minced. Leave the processor running, then drizzle in the oil in a slow, steady stream. Taste the pesto and add more salt and pepper if you think it needs it.

OPTION

• Want pesto for a pasta dish? Add another ¼ cup oil to thin it out a bit.

CHICKPEA BLINTZES *with* CASHEW SOUR CREAM, APPLES, *and* DILL

I first started playing around with this combo in 2005 at a vegan bistro called Counter in New York City. Later, I served it in a larger crepe form with roasted mushrooms, spinach, and aioli as a brunch item in my SAF Restaurant in London. The base is a gluten-free crepe made with chickpea flour. Larger versions of the crepe, also known as crispy chickpea bread, are called *farinata* in Italy and *socca* in France. But I like to make them into little blintzes and top them with cashew sour cream and apples. —*CHAD*

🥄 **SERVES 10 TO 12 AS PASSED CANAPÉS, OR 4 AS LARGER CREPES**

BLINTZES

1½ cups water

1¼ cups chickpea flour

⅓ cup everyday olive oil

1 teaspoon sea salt

Lots of cracked black pepper

Spray oil

TOPPINGS

2 small green apples, such as Granny Smith

1 tablespoon fresh lemon juice

Cashew Sour Cream (page 77)

Dill feathers or flowers, for garnish

1 **FOR THE BLINTZES:** Pour half (¾ cup) of the water into a blender (preferably high-speed) and add the flour, oil, salt, and pepper. Start blending, and when it's mostly smooth, about a minute, slowly add the remaining ¾ cup water until the mixture reaches the consistency of thin pancake batter.

2 Pour the batter into a plastic squeeze bottle, then cut the tip of the cap so the opening is about ¼ inch in diameter.

3 Place a crepe pan or nonstick sauté pan over medium heat and coat with spray oil. When the pan is hot, squeeze 1½- to 2-inch rounds of batter all around the pan. When the batter begins to bubble around the edges, about 2 minutes, flip each blintz. Cook until firm, about 1 minute longer. You may need to do a test batch and adjust the heat to avoid burning. Repeat, stacking the blintzes as you make them. Serve warm, as these blintzes get mealy when they cool.

4 **FOR THE TOPPINGS:** Core the apples, cut in half lengthwise, then shave into paper-thin slices on a mandoline or truffle shaver. Toss with the lemon juice to prevent browning.

5 Spoon some cashew sour cream on each blintz. To get fancy, use two spoons to mold the sour cream into a quenelle (football shape).

6 Place a slice or two of apple on the sour cream. Garnish with dill feathers or flowers.

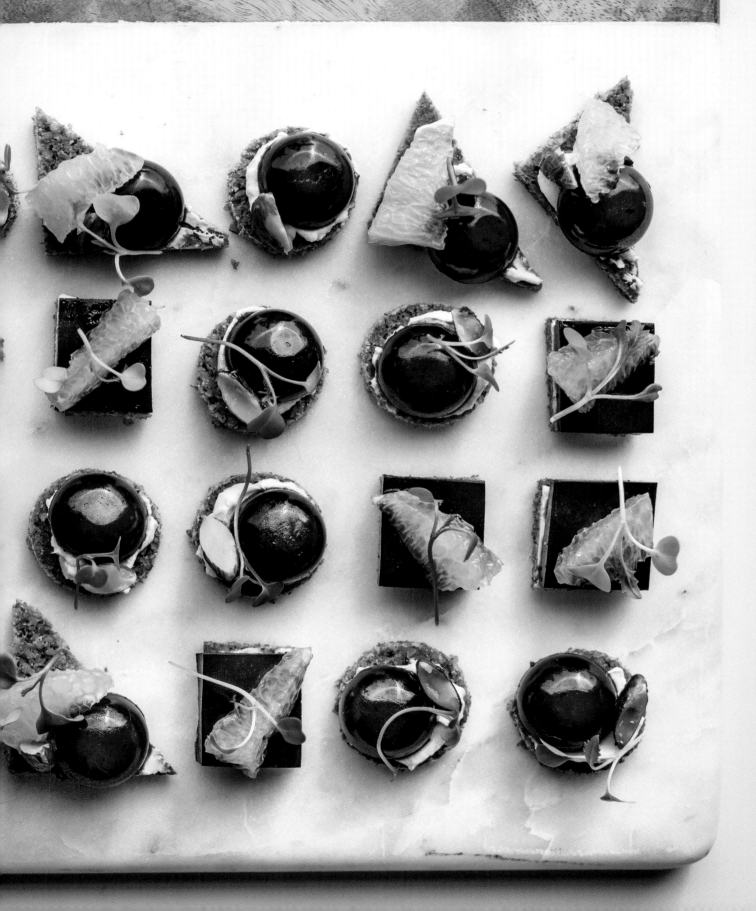

SMOKED TOFU DUMPLINGS *with* SPINACH, DATES, *and* BLACK VINAIGRETTE

I was fortunate to work with Chef David Bailey—a badass kitchen ninja, head chef at my SAF Restaurant in London, and close friend. David makes incredible Pan-Asian food, and he wowed me with a version of these spinach and date dumplings. It's an unusual combination that totally works. I like it even better with a little smoked tofu for protein and earthiness. A drizzle of black vinaigrette gives the dumplings a sharp, malty taste that balances the sweet, savory, and spicy notes in the filling. This one is totally worth the effort. —*CHAD*

SERVES 6 TO 8 (25 TO 35 DUMPLINGS)

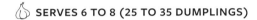

4 cups fresh spinach leaves

½ cup water chestnuts

1 block (6 to 8 ounces) smoked or baked tofu (see Pro Tips, page 86), cubed

¼ cup minced pitted dates

2 tablespoons sherry vinegar

1 tablespoon toasted sesame oil

2 cloves garlic, minced

1 tablespoon minced fresh ginger

1 teaspoon minced red chile (leave out the seeds for less heat)

½ teaspoon sea salt

1 to 1½ packages (12 ounces each) round eggless dumpling skins, about 3½-inch diameter (see Pro Tips, page 86)

1 tablespoon cornstarch

Spray oil for cooking

Cabbage leaves or bamboo leaves, optional

½ cup Black Vinaigrette (page 86)

1 To make the filling, set a steam basket over simmering water in a pan. Put the spinach in the steamer, cover, and steam just until the spinach wilts, 2 to 3 minutes. Transfer to a colander and press water from the spinach. Finely chop, then transfer to a medium mixing bowl.

2 Pulse the water chestnuts in a food processor until coarsely chopped. Add the cubed tofu and pulse a few more times until everything is finely chopped, but not pureed to a mush. Add to the mixing bowl with the spinach, along with the dates, vinegar, sesame oil, garlic, ginger, chile, and salt. Mix thoroughly, making sure that the dates are evenly distributed.

3 To assemble the dumplings, set the bowl of filling, a small cup of water, your dumpling skins, and a baking sheet on a work surface. Scatter some cornstarch over a large baking sheet (to help keep the dumplings from sticking to the pan).

4 For each dumpling, dip your finger in the water and moisten the entire edge of the dumpling (image A). Mound about a tablespoon of filling in the center of the dumpling skin and gently fold it like a taco in your palm (image B). Starting at one corner, crimp the edge of the dumpling skin that is facing you, pressing against the back side that is flat (image C). Continue crimping around the edge of the dumpling to enclose and seal in the filling (image D). You should have enough filling for 25 to 35 dumplings.

RECIPE CONTINUES →

and moisten the entire edge of the dumpling skin. For a shumai-style fold, bring all the sides up to the top and twist gently to make a small round purse. Pinch just under the top opening of the purse to gently close it. You should have enough filling to make 30 to 40 dumplings.

7 These dumplings are best steamed: Spray a steamer basket with oil or line with cabbage leaves or bamboo leaves to prevent sticking. Put the dumplings in the steamer in batches, place over simmering water, cover, and steam until the dumplings are tender, about 3 minutes.

8 Gather 6 to 8 small serving bowls and place 4 or 5 dumplings in the center of each. Pour about ¼ cup broth around the dumplings in each bowl so a little broth comes up the sides of the dumplings. Anoint each bowl with a few drops of chile oil and a couple of basil leaves (or sliced green onions).

Pro Tip

Look for freeze-dried corn in the grain aisle of your market. We're partial to the taste and texture of Karen's Naturals freeze-dried corn. If you can't find it, the recipe works fine without the freeze-dried corn— it's just a little lighter on corn flavor.

LION'S MANE STEAKS

Lion's mane mushrooms rock! They are my favorite—and the meatiest—of all mushrooms. They look soft and fluffy like white pom poms (another name for them). When you press and sear them in a hot pan, they get dense and meaty, nice and brown, and infinitely tastier. Just season them and put them on a plate! For something creamy, spoon on some Cauliflower Mornay Sauce (page 262). Or serve them as sliders in buns with your favorite barbecue sauce. Lion's mane mushrooms are wicked good for you. Research shows that they can help regenerate nerves and improve cognitive function. Brain food! —DEREK

SERVES 4

---

3 tablespoons grapeseed oil or other mild-tasting oil

1 tablespoon plant-based butter

1 pound lion's mane mushrooms (5 or 6 pieces)

1 teaspoon granulated onion

1 teaspoon sea salt

½ teaspoon freshly ground black pepper

1 Heat a large heavy pan (such as cast iron) over medium heat until very hot, about 2 minutes. Add half the oil and half the butter, swirling to coat the pan. Add as many mushrooms as will fit into the pan. Use a second heavy pan or a couple of foil-wrapped bricks to weight down and press/sear the mushrooms. Cook for 2 minutes, then remove the weight and transfer the mushrooms to a work surface.

2 Add the remaining oil and butter to the pan, swirling to coat. Flip the mushrooms and season the cooked side with half of the granulated onion, salt, and pepper. Return the mushrooms to the hot pan, raw-side down. Return the weight to the mushrooms and press/sear the other side for 2 minutes. Remove the weight and flip the mushrooms in the pan.

Season the newly cooked side with the remaining seasonings.

3 Return the weight to the mushrooms and cook another 2 minutes. Repeat this process of flipping, weighting down, and searing the mushrooms until they are condensed and pressed, crispy and golden brown with almost no liquid left in the pan, about 10 minutes total. Poke the mushrooms to test whether they are finished cooking. They should feel compact yet fleshy, the way the fleshy base of your thumb feels when you poke it while firmly making the okay sign.

> **Pro Tip**
> *If you can't find lion's mane mushrooms, use cremini or portobello mushrooms instead. Just remove the stems.*

OPTION

- To barbecue the pressed mushrooms, follow the directions in Barbecued Maitake Steaks (page 223).

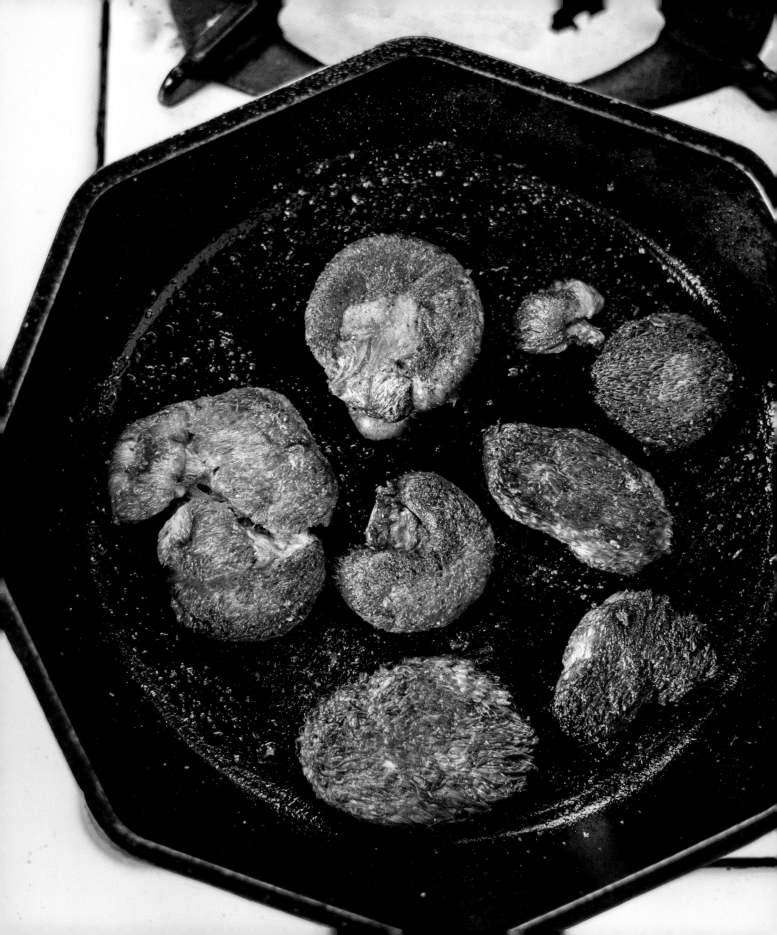

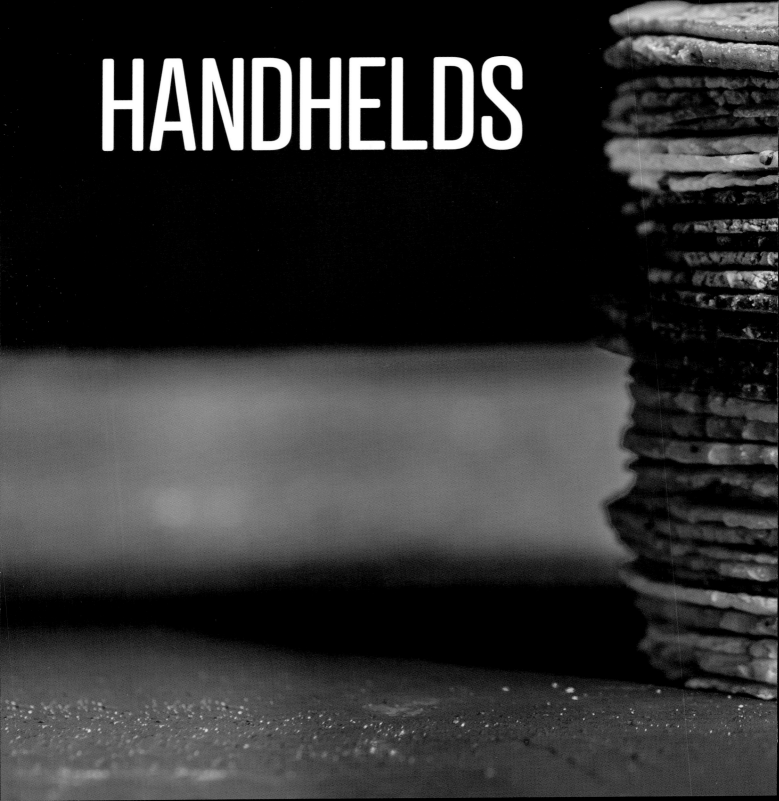

HANDHELDS

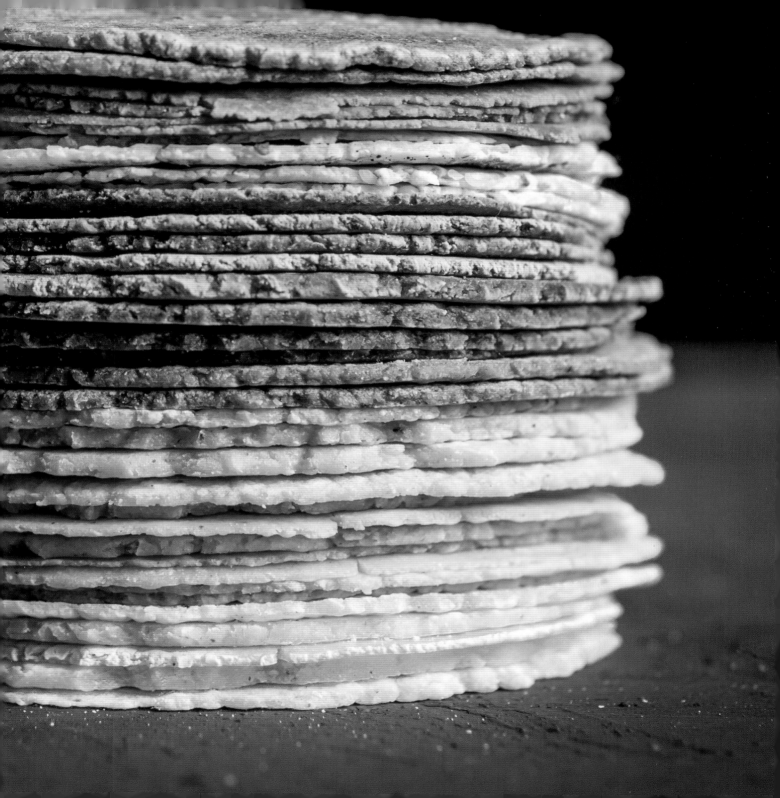

SOURDOUGH STARTER

This recipe and the Sourdough Pizza Dough (page 96) come from our friend Sean Coyne. Sean's baking credits include several years as head baker at Jim Lahey's Sullivan Street Bakery and director of Thomas Keller's bread program at Per Se. Sean is a total pro. This sourdough starter works because organic, unbleached flour (especially rye flour) contains a variety of different natural, wild yeasts and bacterial spores. Just mix in some water and that moisture encourages them to grow. After a few days, the yeast and beneficial bacteria naturally propagate in the flour, and that's your bread starter. Then you feed it fresh flour and water to help it grow stronger. Keep in mind that weight measurements are much more accurate than volumes. If you run into any trouble, make sure you're measuring by weight.

 MAKES 2 TO 2½ CUPS (ABOUT 385 G)

¼ cup (25 g) unbleached unbromated whole-grain rye flour

2¾ cups (345 g) unbleached unbromated all-purpose flour (wheat flour)

1⅓ cups (320 g) warm (about 90°F) water

1 DAYS 1 TO 3: Combine the rye flour, a generous ¾ cup (105 g) all-purpose flour, and about 9 tablespoons (158 g) warm water in a medium bowl. (A glass bowl is best so you can see bubbles forming through the side.) Mix with your hands; this is to capture the yeast, bacteria, and microorganisms from your hands, which will help the sourdough ferment and grow. Mix just until all the flour is wet. The mixture should be somewhat liquid, like loose pancake batter. Let sit, uncovered, at room temperature for 3 to 4 days, stirring now and then. The consistency should still be like liquid pancake batter, but with bubbles. (The bubbles mean that the yeast is active and giving off carbon dioxide.)

2 DAY 4: Throw away all but about 1 tablespoon (9 g) of this liquid starter. (Or, to keep the remaining liquid starter active, see the Options.) By hand, mix 4¾ tablespoons (72 g) warm water into the 1 tablespoon starter, breaking it up with your hands. Add about ½ cup (60 g) all-purpose flour and continue mixing by hand until the mixture comes together. This process feeds and refreshes the liquid starter. Let this new liquid mixture ferment for 12 to 18 hours at room temperature.

3 DAY 5: Remove a generous 2 tablespoons (27 g) of this stiff starter to another mixing bowl. (To keep the remaining stiff starter active, see the Options.) Mix about 6 tablespoons (90 g) warm water into the 2 tablespoons of starter, breaking it up by hand. Add a scant 1½ cups (180 g) all-purpose flour and continue mixing until stiff. The starter should be so stiff that it's difficult to mix in the flour. Let this stiff starter ferment for 12 to 18 hours. At that point, you will be ready to mix up pizza dough and still have enough stiff starter left over to make more dough later.

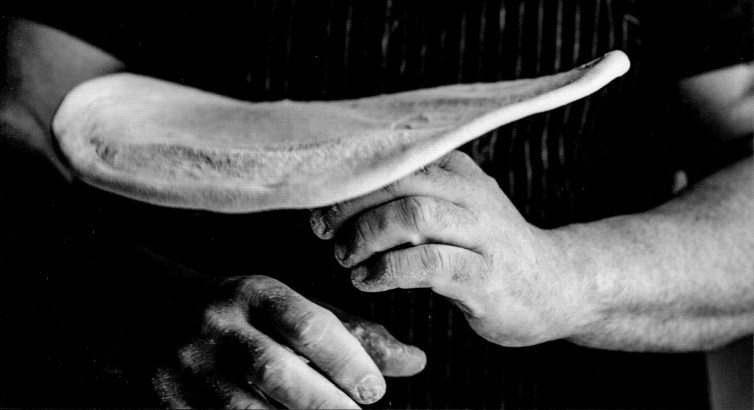
BADASS BAKER, SEAN COYNE

OPTIONS

- You can keep the liquid starter from Day 4 going by feeding it, which allows you to always have starter on hand to make other yeast breads. To keep a small amount of the liquid starter going, follow the directions under Day 4, but instead of throwing away all the excess, put a generous 1 teaspoon (4.5 g) liquid starter in a small bowl. Mix in 2½ tablespoons (36 g) warm water and a scant ¼ cup (30 g) all-purpose flour. Leave the starter out at room temperature and refresh every day, using these same amounts. Or, put in the fridge and refresh it with the same amounts twice a week. You can keep the starter going forever, at either room temperature or in the refrigerator, as long as you keep feeding it.

- You can also keep the stiffer starter from Day 5 going by feeding it. That allows you to mix up breads like Rustic Walnut Bread and Garlic Knots (page 98) in addition to pizza. To keep a small amount of the stiff starter going, follow the directions under Day 5, but instead of throwing away all the excess, put about 1¼ teaspoons (5 g) of the stiff starter in a small bowl. Mix it with 3¼ teaspoons (16 g) warm water and 4¼ tablespoons (33 g) all-purpose flour. Leave the starter out at room temperature and refresh every day, using these same amounts. Or, put in the fridge and refresh it with the same amounts twice a week. You can keep the stiff starter going forever if you keep feeding it.

SOURDOUGH PIZZA DOUGH

If you have an active bread starter, you can use it here in place of our sourdough starter. If using our starter, it should be ready to mix into pizza dough on Day 6 (after fermenting 12 to 18 hours on Day 5). On that day, mix up the pizza dough in the morning and, by midday, the dough will be ready to shape and bake into pizza for lunch. Or you can chill your dough ball and bake the pizza later that evening. So if you're starting from scratch without commercial yeast, you should be able to mix up the starter one weekend, and then bake pizza the following weekend. Most of that time you just let the fermentation happen. The total hands-on time is only about 45 minutes.

 MAKES ABOUT 2¼ POUNDS (1 KG) DOUGH, ENOUGH FOR FOUR 12-INCH PIZZAS

3⅓ cups (420 g) unbleached, unbromated all-purpose flour

1½ cups (360 g) cool (about 65°F) water

1 cup (210 g) stiff Sourdough Starter (page 94)

1¾ teaspoons (10 g) fine sea salt

1   TO MIX: Put the flour, water, and starter in the bowl of an electric mixer fitted with the dough hook. Mix on low speed for 1 minute. It will look loose and shaggy. Scatter salt over the mixture and let everything sit at room temperature for 30 to 45 minutes.

2   Set the mixer to medium-low speed and mix until the dough comes together, 3 to 7 minutes, depending on your mixer. If you have an instant-read thermometer, take the dough's temperature: It should be 75°F to 78°F. If it's greater or less than that, adjust the water temperature the next time you make dough.

3   TO FOLD: Lightly oil a large bowl and scrape the dough into the bowl. To create structure in the dough, fold it: This takes about 10 seconds; simply dig one of your hands underneath the dough, lift it up, and gently stretch the dough until it feels like it's resisting (maybe 6-inch stretching), then fold the stretched part back onto the dough. It should feel loose since this is the first set of folding. Turn the bowl a quarter turn, then stretch and fold again. Repeat, turning the bowl and stretching and folding different parts of the dough four or five times, then invert the dough in the bowl so the folded parts are underneath.

4   Repeat folding the dough like this once every ½ hour for 3 hours. After the last fold, wait 20 minutes before you divide the dough. At that point, the dough should have developed more gluten, feel fuller and puffy, and be ready to roll into a ball.

5   TO ROLL INTO A BALL: For 12-inch pizzas, divide the dough into four equal pieces—each should weigh about 250 g. Very lightly flour your hands and a work surface—not too much because you want the dough to stick so you can stretch it. Imagine the piece of dough in front of you is a half-full water balloon. Use your hands to drag the balloon to one side, tightening

RECIPE CONTINUES →

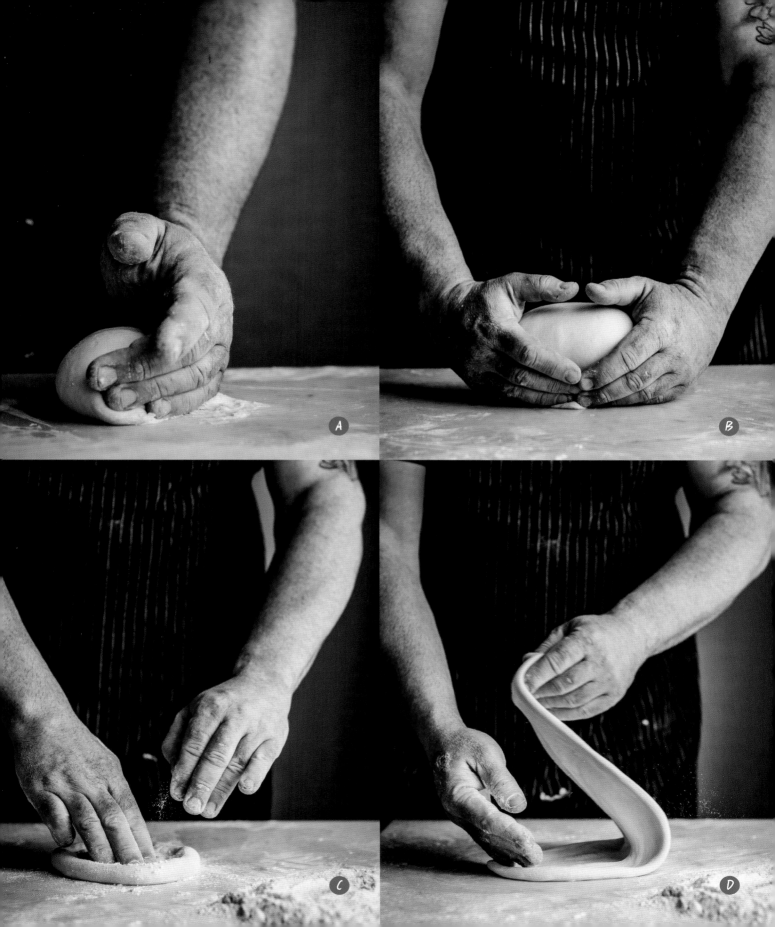

it so it fills with air and swells up on that side (page 97, image A). Use the friction on the work surface to drag and stretch the dough. When the balloon is full, fold the thinner edge of the dough underneath (page 97, image B). Repeat this process a few times, dragging the dough and folding the edges underneath until you have gone all around the outer edges of the dough. At that point, you should have a nice round, smooth ball of dough, maybe with some folds underneath. Don't worry if it's not perfect. Let the dough rest for 1 hour at room temperature before shaping. Or cover it and chill for up to 24 hours, then warm at room temp for 30 minutes before shaping.

6 Crank your oven on full bore, usually 500°F for home ovens. If you have convection, turn it on. If using a baking stone, put it on a rack in the center of the oven. You'll need the broiler later, so if it's on the roof of the oven, position the top rack 4 to 5 inches from the broiler. (If you have a separate broiler— sometimes beneath the oven floor—no need for the top rack.) If using a cast-iron pan, set one rack in the center, and then one rack 4 to 5 inches from the broiler, if it's at the top of the oven.

7 **TO SHAPE:** For a classic 12-inch round pizza with a rim, lightly flour your work surface again, then invert one dough ball onto it. Poke your fingers around the edge of the ball to begin creating a rim (page 97, image C). Then poke your fingers around the center to begin stretching the dough, keeping the rim you just made. Now put one hand gently on top of the dough to secure it, then grab the rim gently with your other hand and stretch it away from the center, picking up the dough slightly as you go (page 97, image D). Repeat stretching all around the edge of the rim until you have a nice 12-inch circle of dough. It goes faster if you pick up the dough and stretch it by draping and rotating it over the backs of your hands, but that takes some practice. Use immediately. Or, to freeze the shaped dough, lightly

oil a plastic bag and seal the dough in it; freeze for up to 1 week and thaw before topping and baking.

8 **TO BAKE ON A BAKING STONE:** Put the stretched dough on a lightly floured pizza peel or rimless baking sheet. Top the pizza, then slide it onto the hot baking stone. When fully risen and the rim starts to brown, after 5 to 7 minutes, use the peel to transfer the pizza under the broiler. Broil until the pizza is blistered and charred in a few spots, 1 to 2 minutes. Transfer the pizza to the oven floor to crisp up the bottom crust, 5 to 10 seconds, depending on the heat of your oven floor.

9 **TO BAKE IN A CAST-IRON PAN:** Heat a large (12- to 14-inch) cast-iron skillet on the stovetop over medium heat. Slide the stretched dough into the hot skillet, then turn the burner to low. Quickly top the pizza, then put the pan of pizza in the oven and bake until the rim browns lightly, 5 to 7 minutes. Move the pan under the broiler and broil until blistered and charred, 1 to 2 minutes.

OPTIONS

RUSTIC WALNUT BREAD: Add 1½ cups toasted chopped walnuts to the fully mixed dough. Fold and rest as directed. Shape into a round or oval loaf, and bake at 400°F for about 30 minutes.

GARLIC KNOTS: Portion half the dough into 12 pieces about 50 g each. Gently cook 5 thinly sliced garlic cloves in 1 cup olive oil over low heat until mellowed in taste but not browned, about 15 minutes. Lightly oil a 12-cup muffin tin with olive oil. Roll each piece of dough into a rope that is 7 to 9 inches long. Tie in a single or double knot and place in the oiled muffin cups. Top each with about 1 tablespoon of the garlic oil mixture; add some red pepper flakes if you like. Let proof (rise) at room temperature until doubled in bulk, about 1 hour. Bake in a 400°F oven until golden brown, about 20 minutes.

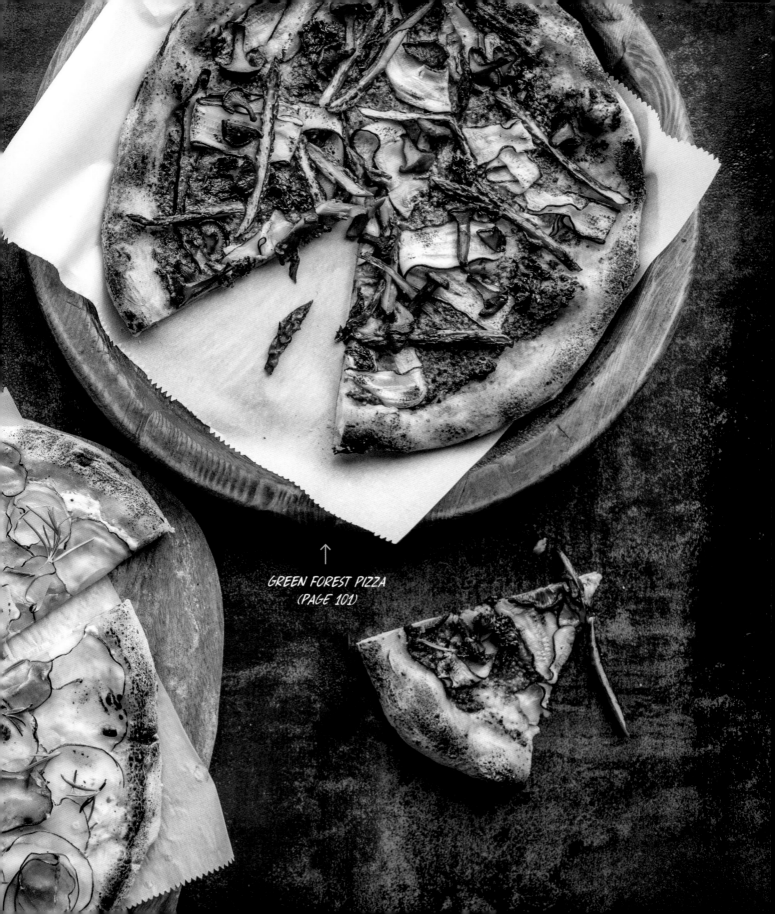

GREEN FOREST PIZZA
(PAGE 101)

FRESH CORN TORTILLAS

It's an incredible feeling to make something yourself that you're used to buying. It's so liberating. Once you start making fresh tortillas, you'll never look back. It's a world of difference in flavor from pre-made tortillas, and they only take 20 minutes to make on any given taco Tuesday. If you mix up the dough in the morning, you can press tortillas out at night in even less time. Or make the dough the night before, and then press the next day. I learned the basics from a cook in Austin years ago, and she turned me on to Gold Mine organic masa harina flour. It has a coarse texture that feels really good in your mouth. Look for white, yellow, and blue corn varieties online or at food co-ops. Sometimes, I like to mix it 50:50 with the more popular Maseca masa harina, which has a finer texture. —CHAD

👄 MAKES 8 TO 10 SMALL TORTILLAS

1 cup fine white masa harina flour, such as from Gold Mine or Maseca

½ teaspoon sea salt, preferably flake salt for crunch

About 1 cup warm water

Spray oil, for the pan

1 Mix the flour and salt by hand in a mixing bowl. Drizzle in the warm water in ¼-cup increments, mixing well. (Warm water hydrates the dough faster than cold water and helps you get the right moistness.) The dough should feel soft and a little grainy, like slightly wet Play-Doh. When you roll the finished dough between your palms, you should see a light speckle of masa grains on your skin. Add just enough water to get to that consistency. If adding wet ingredients (see the Options, page 106), such as vegetable purees, herbs, or liquid extracts, you won't need quite as much water. If adding dry ingredients such as spices, other flours, or seeds, you'll need a little extra water.

2 Gather the dough into a ball and place in a zipper-lock bag. Let it rest for 15 to 20 minutes to hydrate the masa. You can also refrigerate the dough ball in a zipper-lock bag for a few days (see Pro Tip).

3 When you're ready to cook some tortillas, heat a heavy pan over medium heat. (I like to use a large cast-iron griddle over two burners so I can cook 3 or 4 tortillas at a time.) Spray or coat the pan with oil, then wipe with a paper towel to leave only a thin film of oil on the pan.

4 Get a new gallon-size zipper-lock bag and cut off the zipper top. Cut down the two opposite sides, so you are left with a folded piece of plastic with a crease. This is your nonstick surface for pressing tortillas.

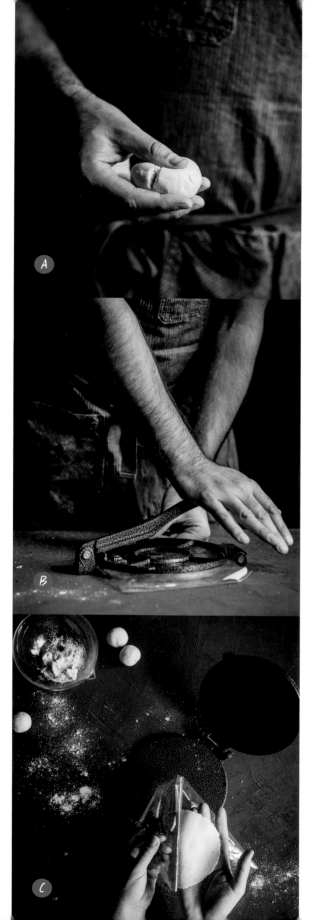

A

B

C

5 Roll the dough into balls the size of Ping-Pong balls, about 1½ inches in diameter (image A). Place a ball on one half of the plastic, cover with the other half, and flatten slightly with your palm. Place on a tortilla press, and press gently (image B). Tortilla presses vary in width, so rotate the tortilla a few times, pressing the dough to about an ⅛-inch thickness.

6 Gently peel off the plastic (image C), place the tortilla on the hot pan, and cook for about 30 seconds. Be patient and resist the temptation to touch it. When the edges look slightly dry and splintered with teeny cracks, after about 30 seconds or 1 minute, use a spatula to flip the tortilla; cook for 20 seconds more. Repeat one or two more times to get a little bit of color on your tortilla. Transfer to a tortilla warmer or clean kitchen towel, allowing the tortilla to steam and soften for 10 minutes or so. Gentle steaming is important. If you use fresh tortillas right away without steaming, they're more likely to crack. Keep pressing, cooking, and stacking/steaming tortillas, re-using the zipper-lock bag. Use immediately or keep covered at room temperature for a few hours.

Pro Tip
To keep the tortillas for a couple of days in the fridge, add 1½ teaspoons cornstarch to the dough. Cornstarch will make the tortillas more pliable so they're less likely to crack when chilled.

RECIPE CONTINUES →

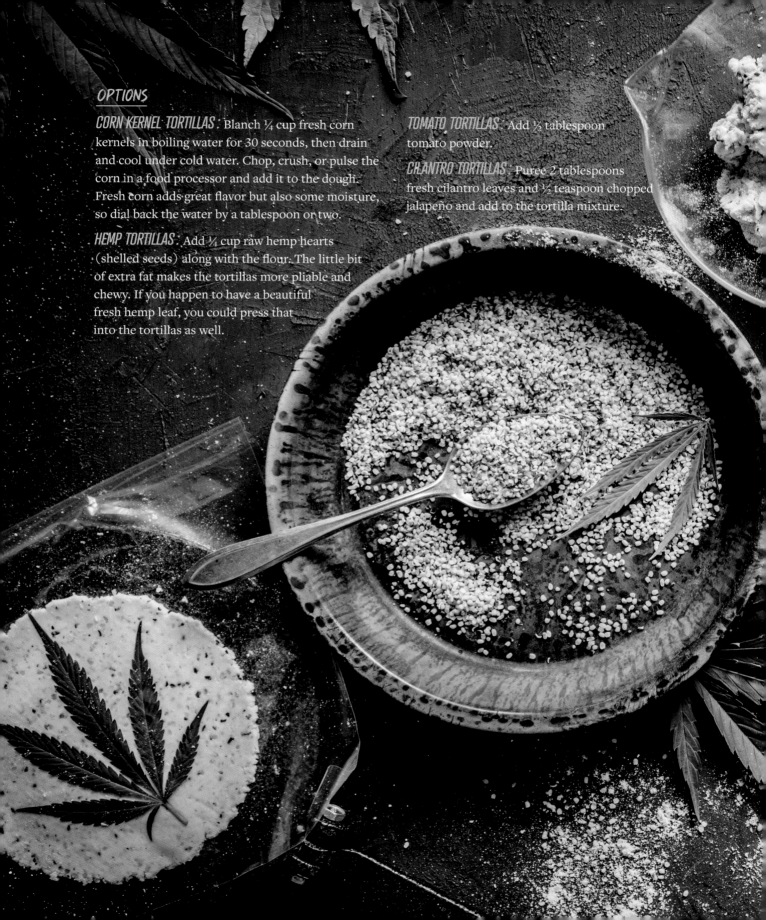

OPTIONS

CORN KERNEL TORTILLAS: Blanch ¼ cup fresh corn kernels in boiling water for 30 seconds, then drain and cool under cold water. Chop, crush, or pulse the corn in a food processor and add it to the dough. Fresh corn adds great flavor but also some moisture, so dial back the water by a tablespoon or two.

HEMP TORTILLAS: Add ¼ cup raw hemp hearts (shelled seeds) along with the flour. The little bit of extra fat makes the tortillas more pliable and chewy. If you happen to have a beautiful fresh hemp leaf, you could press that into the tortillas as well.

TOMATO TORTILLAS: Add ⅓ tablespoon tomato powder.

CILANTRO TORTILLAS: Puree 2 tablespoons fresh cilantro leaves and ½ teaspoon chopped jalapeño and add to the tortilla mixture.

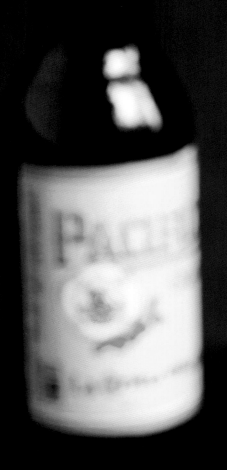

Pro Tip

Lion's mane mushrooms usually pop up in the fall. If you can't find them, use 2 portobello mushrooms, remove the stems, then scrape the gills from the underside of the caps. Peel the tops of the caps to make them as flat as possible, and then proceed with the recipe.

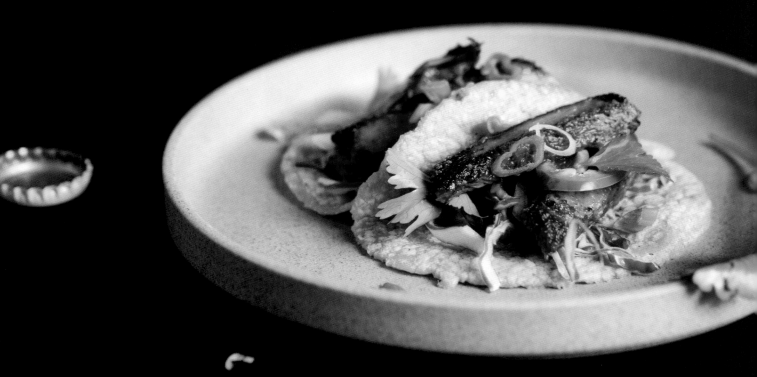

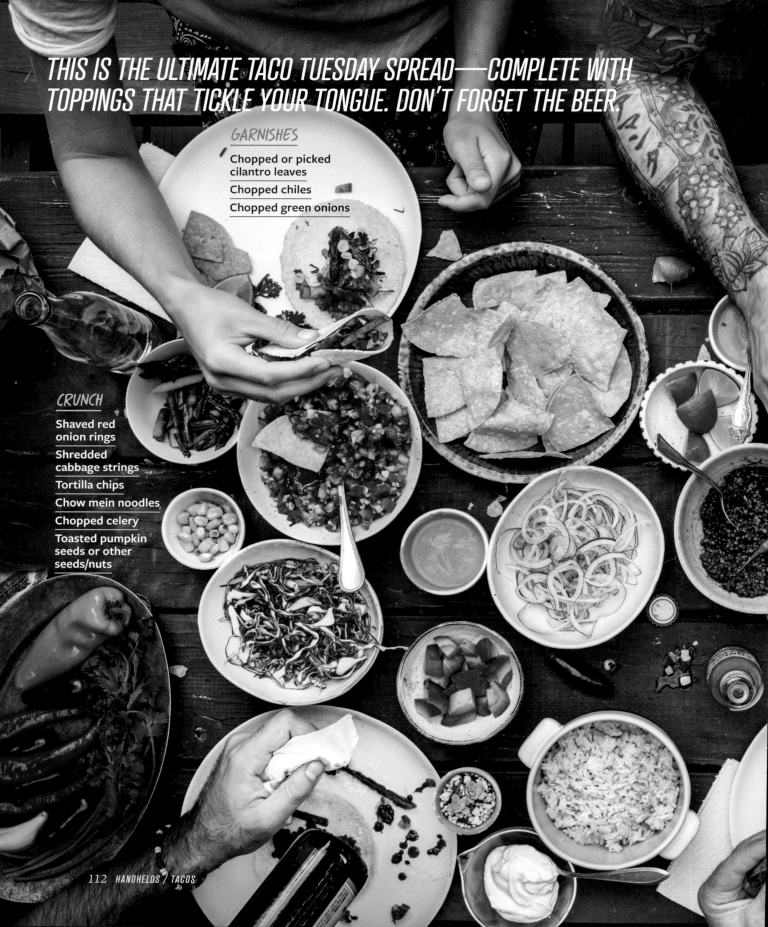

THIS IS THE ULTIMATE TACO TUESDAY SPREAD—COMPLETE WITH TOPPINGS THAT TICKLE YOUR TONGUE. DON'T FORGET THE BEER.

GARNISHES

Chopped or picked cilantro leaves

Chopped chiles

Chopped green onions

CRUNCH

Shaved red onion rings

Shredded cabbage strings

Tortilla chips

Chow mein noodles

Chopped celery

Toasted pumpkin seeds or other seeds/nuts

TACO BAR with TACO TICKLERS

BASES

Fresh Corn Tortillas (page 104) or store-bought

Hot Chocolate Lentils (page 108)

Cooked beans

Cooked rice or grains

FOCAL POINTS

Barbecued Maitake Steaks (page 223)

Lion's Mane Carne Asada (page 110)

Grilled asparagus

Grilled mushrooms

CREAMY

Diced avocado or guacamole

Cashew Sour Cream (page 77) or Kite Hill yogurt

Follow Your Heart shredded cheddar

Wicked Healthy Cheese Sauce (page 260)

ACID/KICK

Poached Corn Salsa (page 275)

Heirloom Tomato Salsa (page 274) and/or hot sauce

Creamy Jalapeño Salsa (page 273)

Carrot Habanero Citrus Hot Sauce (page 278)

Quick Pickled Vegetables (page 279) or kimchi

Cut limes or other citrus, for squeezing

JACKFRUIT CARNITAS TACOS

Fruit tacos? Not quite. Here, we're talking about green, unripe jackfruit, which tastes savory, almost like mushrooms without the earthiness. It's pretty amazing. The best thing, though, is the texture. It stays firm and chewy when cooked and shreds up just like pulled pork. Boom—plant-based carnitas! I rarely use canned food, but jackfruit works. Most Asian markets sell brined green jackfruit in cans, and health food stores often carry green jackfruit in vacuum-pack pouches. Look for unseasoned jackfruit from the Jackfruit Company or Upton's Naturals. Then season, braise, and serve in tortillas with your favorite taco adornments. Yum! —*CHAD*

🍋 SERVES 4

JACKFRUIT AND SPICE RUB

3 cups green jackfruit (from a pouch), drained and rinsed

3 cloves garlic, minced

½ teaspoon paprika

½ teaspoon granulated onion

½ teaspoon freshly ground black pepper

¼ teaspoon ground chipotle pepper

¼ teaspoon ground coriander

¼ teaspoon ground cinnamon

Sea salt to taste

BRAISING LIQUID

2½ tablespoons everyday olive oil

1 medium onion, diced

1 cup Vegetable Stock (page 284) or store-bought

¼ cup orange juice

1 lime, juiced

2 tablespoons maple syrup

1½ teaspoons minced fresh oregano

2 bay leaves

1 chipotle chile in adobo sauce, minced

Sea salt to taste

ASSEMBLY

8 to 10 Fresh Corn Tortillas (page 104) or store-bought

1½ avocados, pitted, peeled, and sliced

½ cup finely shredded cabbage

Heirloom Tomato Salsa (page 274) or store-bought

½ cup picked cilantro leaves

2 limes, cut into wedges

1 *FOR THE JACKFRUIT AND SPICE RUB:* Cut the inner cores from the drained jackfruit, then slice the cores into strips. (The cores will not shred like the rest of the fruit so you need to slice them.) Place all the jackfruit in a medium bowl.

2 Mix together the garlic, paprika, granulated onion, black pepper, chipotle pepper, coriander, cinnamon, and salt. Sprinkle the spice rub over all of the jackfruit and mix together, roughly shredding the jackfruit. While mixing, pick out any visible seeds. Let marinate in the refrigerator for at least 1 hour or up to overnight.

3 *FOR THE BRAISING LIQUID:* Heat a small Dutch oven or shallow pot over medium-high heat. Add the oil, then the diced onion, and sauté until the onion is golden, 4 to 5 minutes. Add the jackfruit and stir until it begins to stick to the pan, 2 to 3 minutes. Add the stock, stirring to deglaze the pan. Stir in the orange juice, lime juice, maple syrup, oregano, bay leaves, and chipotle. After a minute or two, taste the mixture and season lightly with salt until it tastes good to you. The mixture will cook down later and reduce in volume, so avoid making it too salty.

4 Bring to a simmer, breaking up the jackfruit with a potato masher or fork. Reduce the heat to medium low, cover, and cook until most of the liquid reduces to a sauce that coats the jackfruit, 20 to 25 minutes. Stir frequently to break the jackfruit into shreds and prevent sticking.

5 **TO ASSEMBLE THE TACOS**: Serve the jackfruit on tortillas with avocado, cabbage, salsa, cilantro, and lime wedges for squeezing.

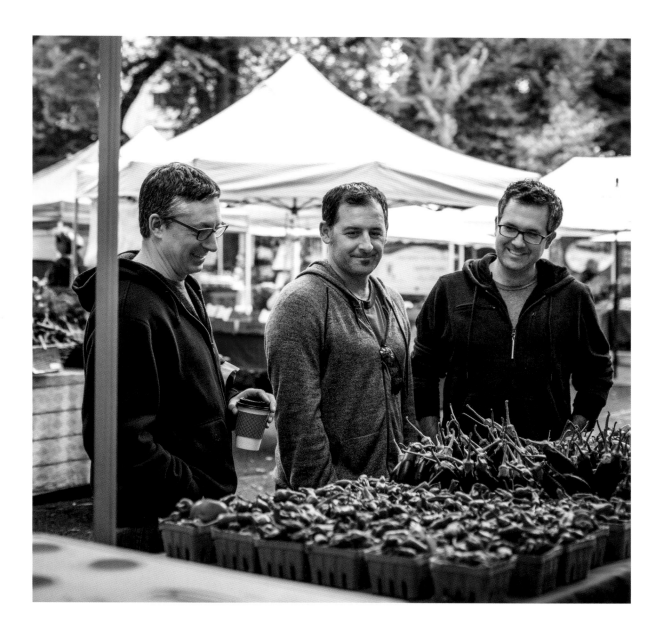

SAMURAI BURGER *with* WASABI, SESAME, CUCUMBER, *and* KIMCHI MAYO

The Beyond Burger from Beyond Meat is a very special plant-based burger. It's thick and satisfying with a super-meaty, umami flavor. Mind-blowing! Here, I take the burger in an Asian direction with kimchi mayo and a crust of sesame seeds, fried garlic, and crushed wasabi peas. But you could go BBQ and blend the kimchi with Smoky BBQ Sauce (page 266) instead of mayo. Or try any of the barbecue sauces on page 224. —*DEREK*

 MAKES 4 BURGERS

⅓ cup wasabi peas

¼ cup fried garlic (see Pro Tip)

½ cup mixed black and white sesame seeds

2 tablespoons plant-based butter

4 soft, squishy hamburger buns

4 Beyond Meat Beyond Burgers (1 pound total)

2 tablespoons tamari or soy sauce

1 tablespoon toasted sesame oil

½ cup Kimchi Mayo (page 117), for garnish

Thinly sliced red onion, crisped up in ice water, for garnish

¼ English cucumber, sliced thin on a diagonal, tossed with 2 tablespoons kimchi liquid, for garnish

Thinly sliced red chiles, for garnish

1 Crush the wasabi peas under a medium cast-iron skillet, then mix them with the fried garlic and sesame seeds in a wide bowl. This is the crust for your burgers.

2 Melt the butter in the skillet over medium heat. Brown the cut sides of the buns in the hot butter, then remove to a work surface.

3 Crank the heat under the skillet to medium high. When wicked hot, add the burgers and cook until seared and browned, 3 to 5 minutes per side.

4 Meanwhile, whisk together the tamari and sesame oil in a wide bowl until blended. Dip the cooked burgers in the tamari mixture, then coat in the sesame seed crust.

5 Pile the burgers onto the buns with the kimchi mayo, red onion, cukes, and chiles.

> **Pro Tip**
> *You can find fried garlic, usually from Thailand, in jars in Asian markets and some grocery stores.*

KIMCHI MAYO (KIMYO)

Try this with the Banh Mi (page 124), too, or as a dip for roasted potatoes.

 MAKES ABOUT 2 CUPS

½ jar (7 ounces) kimchi

½ jar (7 ounces) plant-based mayo, such as Just Mayo

1 tablespoon toasted sesame oil

Blend the kimchi in a blender (preferably high-speed), slowly at first, then gradually speeding up, until the kimchi is smooth. Blend in the mayo and sesame oil until smooth. Keep chilled in the fridge for up to a week.

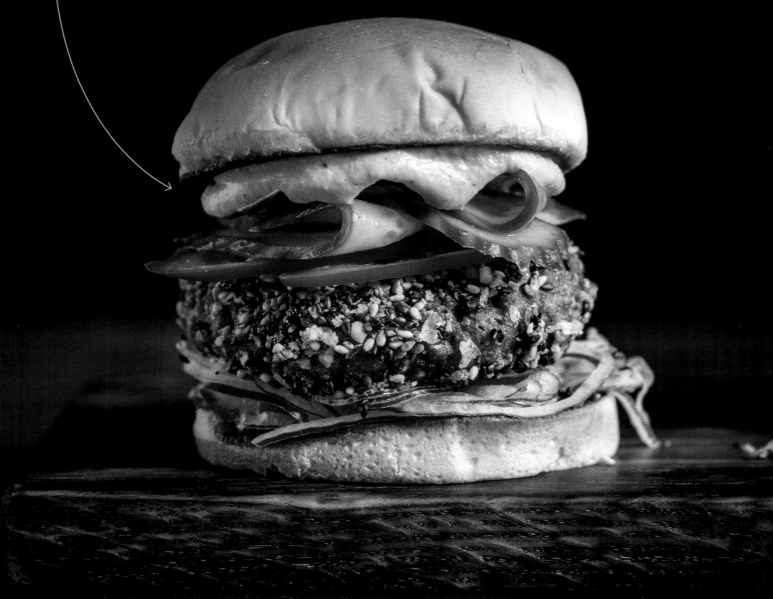

SLOPPY BBQ JACKFRUIT SLIDERS *with* SLAW, SRIRACHA MAYO, *and* PICKLES

Get a roll of paper towels and dive in. Sticky, spicy BBQ sauce, creamy sriracha mayo, crunchy slaw, and sour pickles...this little sandwich has got it going on. And the jackfruit: If you haven't tried it yet, get ready for one of the chewiest, most satisfying plant foods out there. It falls apart in shreds just like you want it to in a sloppy, saucy sandwich. See the headnote to the Jackfruit Carnitas Tacos recipe on page 114 for more info on green jackfruit. —*CHAD*

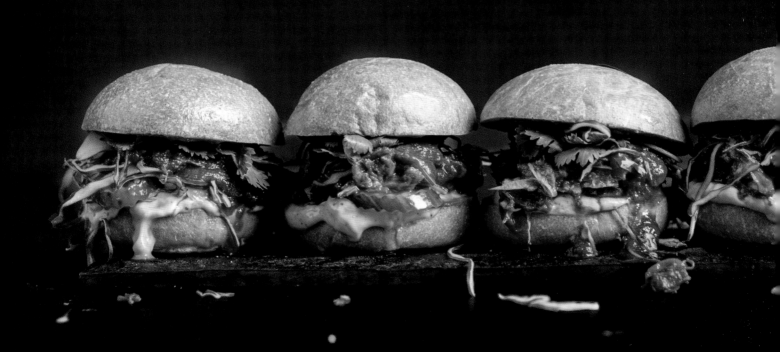

3½ cups green jackfruit (from a pouch), drained and rinsed

3 tablespoons everyday olive oil

1 small white onion, cut into narrow strips

2 cloves garlic, minced

Smoky BBQ Sauce (page 266), prepared through step 3 (i.e., not reduced; see Pro Tip)

½ cup chopped fresh cilantro

3 cups finely shaved green cabbage

USE A MANDOLINE!

½ lime, juiced

Sea salt and freshly ground black pepper

8 to 10 soft, squishy, slider-size buns, toasted if you like

1 cup thin dill pickle rounds

½ cup Sriracha Mayo (page 264)

1 Cut the inner cores from the drained jackfruit, then slice the cores into strips. (The cores will not shred like the rest of the fruit so you need to slice them.)

2 Heat 2 tablespoons of the oil in a sauté pan over medium heat. Add the onion and cook, stirring now and then, until lightly browned, 4 to 6 minutes. Add the jackfruit and cook, stirring a few times, until lightly browned as well, 4 to 6 minutes. This browning process really deepens the flavor of the onions and jackfruit. Add the garlic near the end of the process and cook for just a couple of minutes, until everything is nicely browned.

3 Scrape the jackfruit mixture into the pot of BBQ sauce. Bring everything to a simmer over medium heat, then cut the heat to medium low and simmer gently until the liquid reduces in volume by about one-fourth, 8 minutes or so. Give it a stir now and then to make sure the jackfruit doesn't stick to the pan bottom. You want to reduce the liquid enough so that the jackfruit mixture will sit on a sandwich bun but still be kinda wet and sloppy. When it reaches that consistency, stir in ¼ cup of the cilantro and remove the pot from the heat.

4 To make a quick slaw, toss together the cabbage, lime juice, remaining 1 tablespoon olive oil, and remaining ¼ cup cilantro. Season with salt and pepper, then taste it, adding more seasoning as needed.

5 To assemble, spoon a generous pile of BBQ jackfruit onto each bun and top with pickles, slaw, and a drizzle of sriracha mayo. Sometimes we set everything out and let guests assemble the sammies themselves.

> **Pro Tip**
> *You want to prepare the BBQ sauce up to the point of adding all the ingredients, but don't reduce the liquid yet. This is so that when you add the jackfruit to the sauce and then reduce it, the jackfruit soaks up some of the flavor. You can also use bottled barbecue sauce in this recipe—see the Option.*

OPTION

- To use store-bought barbecue sauce instead of our Smoky BBQ Sauce, put 2 cups of sauce in a large pot and stir in 1 cup Vegetable Stock (page 284), or store-bought, to thin it out a bit. Then add the jackfruit mixture to the pot and simmer it until reduced in volume by one-fourth, proceeding with the recipe as directed.

NEW ENGLAND LOBSTER ROLL

We grew up on the east coast of New Hampshire, where fish 'n' chips, fried clams, and lobster rolls are everywhere. I can still smell the heavy salt air of Hampton Beach and taste the briny, creamy, fresh lobster rolls. When I moved to Portland, Oregon, and lobster mushrooms were everywhere, I decided to reclaim my childhood—plant-pusher style. Lobster mushrooms have a red-orange color that looks just like cooked lobster. They're also super dense and meaty with a mineral flavor reminiscent of lobster. They're perfect for poaching and serving in classic Down East sandwiches, Wicked Healthy style. —*DEREK*

 MAKES 4 ROLLS

4 cups water

¼ cup white miso

2 tablespoons plant-based butter, at room temperature, plus more for buttering the rolls

1¼ teaspoons Old Bay seasoning

1 lemon, halved

2 cups ½-inch chunks cleaned lobster mushrooms (see Pro Tips)

1 kombu strip, about 2 x 4 inches

1 bay leaf

½ cup Plant-Based Mayo (page 264) or store-bought, such as Just Mayo

3 tablespoons diced celery

Coarse sea salt and freshly ground black pepper

4 hot dog rolls, preferably top-sliced, New England style

6 to 8 leaves green leaf lettuce

4 or 5 sprigs fresh flat-leaf parsley, for garnish

1 Combine the water, miso, 2 tablespoons butter, and 1 teaspoon of the Old Bay in a medium saucepan. Squeeze 1 teaspoon lemon juice into the pan, then whisk everything together. Add the mushroom chunks, kombu, and bay leaf and bring almost to a simmer over medium heat. Watch carefully to make sure it does not boil. Boiling kills miso. Don't kill the miso! Just before it simmers, cut the heat to low and simmer very gently to poach the mushrooms, about 30 minutes. Stir now and then to mix the flavors.

2 Use a slotted spoon to remove only the mushroom chunks to a bowl. Cover and chill in the fridge, about 1 hour. (Save the broth in a sealed container for another use; see Pro Tips. It'll keep for weeks in the fridge.)

3 To make the lobster salad, stir together the chilled mushrooms, mayo, celery, 1 teaspoon lemon juice, and remaining ¼ teaspoon Old Bay in a medium bowl. Season with a pinch of salt and pepper if you must.

4 To toast the buns, spread a thin layer of butter evenly on the outside cut sides of each bun. Toast on a griddle or grill over medium heat until golden brown, 2 to 3 minutes per side.

5 Line the toasted buns with lettuce leaves, then fill each with the lobster salad. Garnish with some parsley sprigs. Cut the remaining lemon half into wedges for squeezing.

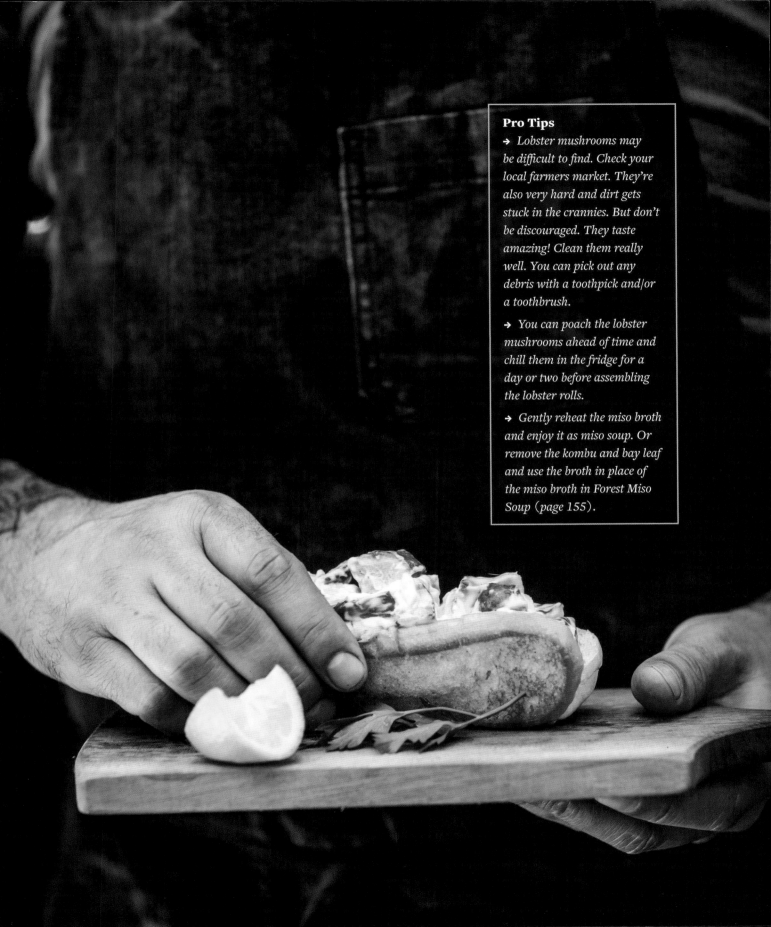

Pro Tips

→ *Lobster mushrooms may be difficult to find. Check your local farmers market. They're also very hard and dirt gets stuck in the crannies. But don't be discouraged. They taste amazing! Clean them really well. You can pick out any debris with a toothpick and/or a toothbrush.*

→ *You can poach the lobster mushrooms ahead of time and chill them in the fridge for a day or two before assembling the lobster rolls.*

→ *Gently reheat the miso broth and enjoy it as miso soup. Or remove the kombu and bay leaf and use the broth in place of the miso broth in Forest Miso Soup* (page 155).

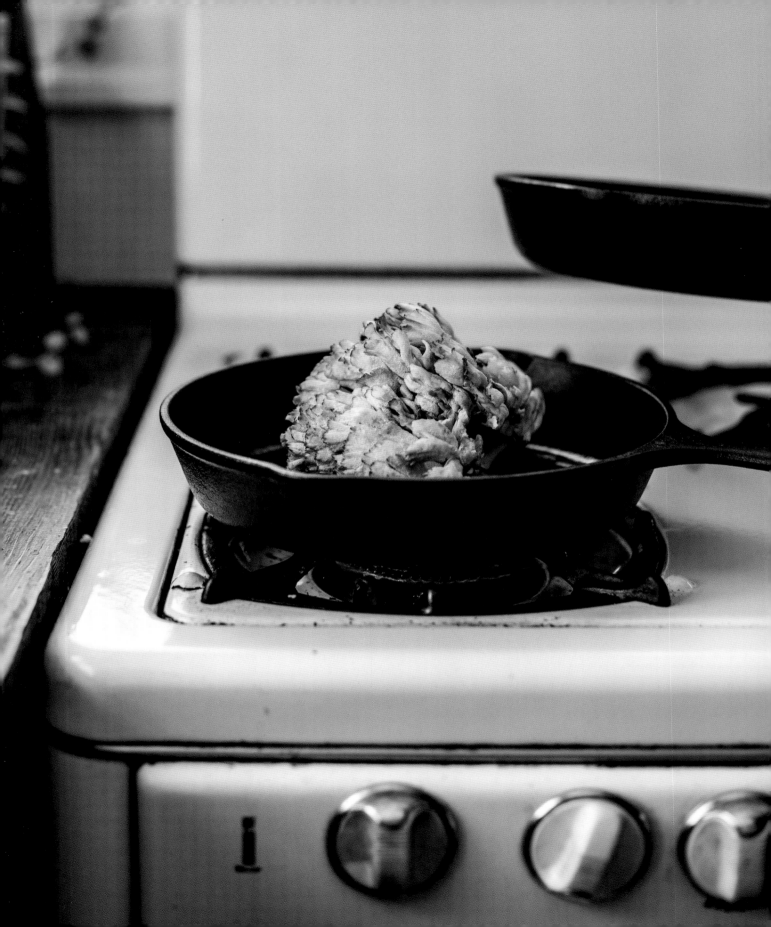

SPICY MAITAKE STEAK SANDWICH

Steak sandwich? Yes, please! You can use any flavor option in the Barbecued Maitake Steak recipe—they are all winners. My favorite is the Bulgogi. What can I say? I have a weakness for Asian flavors. —DEREK

 MAKES 4 SANDWICHES

4 soft sub rolls, each about 6 inches long

½ cup Plant-Based Mayo (page 264) or store-bought, such as Just Mayo

8 slices (8 ounces) plant-based cheese, such as Follow Your Heart pepper jack

½ red onion, sliced thin on a mandoline

Barbecued Maitake Steaks (page 223), sliced thin

4 whole medium dill pickles, sliced on an angle into ovals

½ cup Kimchi Mayo (page 117)

2 jalapeño chiles, sliced thin on an angle

SEED THEM IF YOU LIKE IT MILD

1 cup fresh cilantro and/or mint leaves

1 teaspoon sea salt

1 teaspoon freshly ground black pepper

1 Preheat the oven to 350°F. Cut the sub rolls in half lengthwise, leaving the two halves attached on one side. Place on a baking sheet and spread 1 tablespoon plain mayo on the inside of each half of each roll.

2 Tear each cheese slice in half and lay two halves over the mayo on the rolls. Bake until the rolls are toasted and the cheese melts, 5 to 10 minutes.

3 Meanwhile, soak the sliced onions in ice water for 5 to 10 minutes. (This process tames the sharp bite of the onions and crisps them up a bit. Trust us—it makes them taste better.)

4 To make your sandwiches: Add a layer of the sliced barbecued mushrooms to each roll, then some pickles and onions. Lather on some kimchi mayo, then top with jalapeño, fresh herbs, and salt and pepper. Serve whole or cut in half. To take it with you, wrap it in foil, and grab and go.

Pro Tip

You can slice and sear the maitake steaks a day or two ahead. The kimchi mayo can be made a week ahead and refrigerated.

BANH MI *with* LEMONGRASS TOFU *and* GINGER AIOLI

It drives me bonkers when banh mi are made with stiff-crusted French baguettes. That tough crust rips the roof of your mouth, and the bread's so firm it squishes out the filling. You want soft bread for banh mi. Crispy, but thin crust. That's what a Vietnamese-style baguette is all about, and if you can find it, you'll have yourself a killer sandwich. A hoagie or sub sandwich roll also works. Either way, the bread should lovingly cradle the mix of tart, sweet, salty, spicy, creamy, and crunchy ingredients inside. —CHAD

 MAKES 4 SANDWICHES

BAKED LEMONGRASS TOFU

1 block (14 ounces) extra-firm tofu

½ cup prepared lemonade or orange juice

¼ cup agave syrup

3 tablespoons tamari or soy sauce

3 tablespoons rice vinegar

2 tablespoons thinly sliced lemongrass (use a mandoline)

1 small red chile, sliced into thin rounds

½ tablespoon grated or zested fresh ginger

ASSEMBLY

4 small (6-inch) Vietnamese-style baguettes or sub sandwich rolls

½ cup Ginger Aioli (page 125)

¾ cup Pickled Carrots and Chiles (page 125)

½ avocado, pitted, peeled, and sliced

Handful of fresh cilantro sprigs

A few drizzles of Homemade Badass Sriracha (page 276) or other sriracha

1 **TO BAKE THE TOFU:** Press the tofu like a sandwich between paper towels and plates weighted down with a heavy book. Let it press for at least 10 minutes or up to 1 hour. (Pressing gives tofu a firmer texture and helps it absorb more marinade.)

2 Preheat the oven to 325°F.

3 Slice the pressed slab of tofu lengthwise into 6 to 8 thinner slabs, each about ¼ inch thick. Mix the lemonade, agave, tamari, vinegar, lemongrass, chile, and ginger in a baking dish large enough to hold all the tofu slabs in a single layer (a 13- x 9-inch dish works well). Place the tofu in the marinade and flip each slab to coat completely. Bake for 45 minutes. Use a spatula to carefully flip each slab, then continue baking until the marinade is completely absorbed but not burning, another 20 to 30 minutes. Burning is bad here. Let cool in the baking dish.

4 When cool, cut the tofu diagonally into triangles. This whole process can be done a few days ahead. Just chill the baked tofu triangles in the fridge.

5 **TO ASSEMBLE:** Slice the baguettes or rolls lengthwise to open them up, leaving the two halves attached. For each sandwich, spread a generous amount of aioli on both bread halves. Layer on 3 or 4 slices of tofu, some pickled carrots and chiles, and sliced avocado. Garnish with a few cilantro sprigs and drizzle with sriracha.

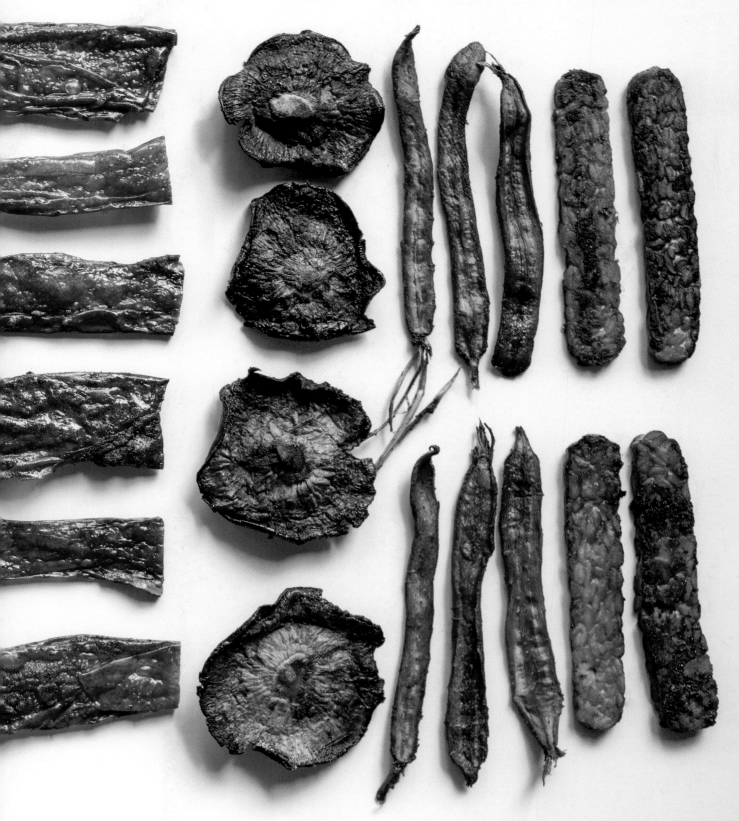

SHIITAKE   CARROT   TEMPEH

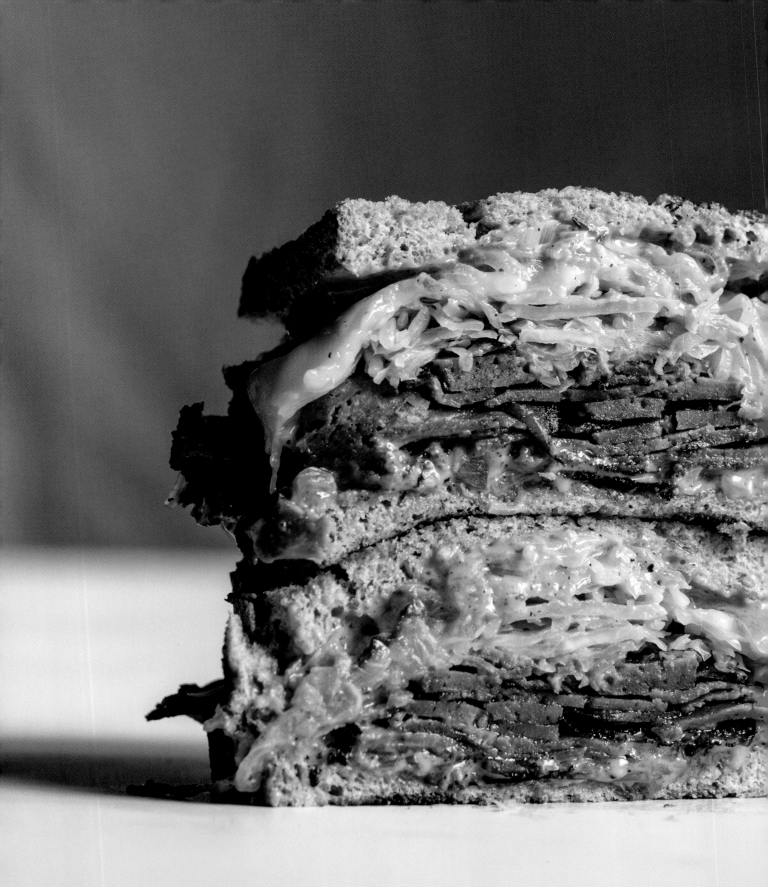

KICKASS PLANT-BASED REUBEN *on* DARK RYE

Whenever I'm in Chicago, I will go out of my way to cross town for the plant-based Reuben at Chicago Diner. It's what dreams are made of. I believe they use pickle juice to flavor the seitan, which gives it the perfect acidity. Crisp seitan, creamy Russian dressing, earthy rye bread, spunky sauerkraut, and soft cheese: I just can't get enough. Here's my version of this comfort food. This is your home-on-Sunday-with-nothing-to-do sandwich. Eat one (or two), flop on the couch, and embrace naptime. —*CHAD*

 MAKES 6 SANDWICHES

SEITAN

2½ cups vital wheat gluten

½ cup chickpea flour

¼ cup nutritional yeast

1 cup Coriander Spice Mix (page 135)

1 cup chopped peeled red beet

1½ cups Vegetable Stock (page 284) or store-bought

⅓ cup dry sherry

3 tablespoons tamari

3 tablespoons tomato paste

2 tablespoons maple syrup

Spray oil

CARAMELIZED ONIONS

1 tablespoon everyday olive oil

2 onions, sliced paper-thin

Sea salt and freshly ground black pepper

ASSEMBLY

1 tablespoon everyday olive oil

1 cup sauerkraut

6 to 8 slices plant-based cheese, such as Chao Field Roast

12 slices dark rye bread, lightly toasted or grilled

1¼ cups Sriracha Russian Dressing (page 264) or store-bought Follow Your Heart Thousand Island

1 TO MAKE THE SEITAN: In a medium bowl, mix together the wheat gluten, chickpea flour, nutritional yeast, and half of the spice mix (½ cup).

2 Put the beets, stock, sherry, tamari, tomato paste, and maple syrup in a blender (preferably high-speed), and blend until very smooth. The consistency will be somewhat thick, like a smoothie.

3 Make a well in the center of the dry ingredients and pour in the blended mixture. Mix well by hand, making sure everything is fully blended together. You'll end up with very stiff Play-Doh-like dough because you are working the gluten and developing its strength. You may need to adjust the wheat gluten and/or vegetable stock up or down to achieve the stiff Play-Doh consistency. Keep mixing until it reaches that consistency.

4 Preheat the oven to 350°F. Coat 2 large pieces of heavy-duty foil with spray oil and set aside.

RECIPE CONTINUES →

5 Roll and stretch the seitan dough to create a log-shaped loaf about 10 inches long and 4 to 5 inches in diameter. The dough will be stiff; just keep working it to create that shape. Transfer the loaf to the foil and coat all over with the remaining spice mix (½ cup), rolling the loaf in the foil for even coating. Roll up the seitan in the foil and wrap it in a tight cylinder. Twist the ends like a Tootsie Roll, then fold in the ends. Make sure it's wrapped tight to keep the seitan from expanding during baking.

6 Place the seitan roll on a baking sheet and bake until extremely firm, turning the roll every 15 to 20 minutes for even cooking. Test the doneness by squeezing it with tongs. The seitan should feel very stiff, like it will be an effort to slice. It will take 80 to 90 minutes to reach this fully cooked texture.

7 Let cool completely in the foil. This is an important step because the seitan will expand and loosen up if you remove it from the foil before cooling. (Weird, right?!)

8 Once fully cooled, the loaf will firm up even more. At that point, you can slice it thin for sandwiches or dice it and brown it for tacos or bowls, or whatever you like. For these Reubens, shave 3 cups paper-thin slices. (You'll have some seitan left over; wrap it and chill for a week or two, or freeze it for a month or so.)

9 *TO CARAMELIZE THE ONIONS:* Heat a large deep sauté pan over medium-high heat. Add the oil, then the onions, and cook for a minute or two. Cut the heat to medium low, cover the pan, and cook, stirring often, until the onions are deeply browned, 15 to 20 minutes. To prevent burning, add a splash of water now and then, scraping up the browned glaze from the pan bottom. Season with salt and pepper, and remove the caramelized onions to a plate.

10 *TO ASSEMBLE EACH SANDWICH:* Heat the same pan over medium-high heat. Add about ½ teaspoon of the oil, then about ½ cup of the shaved seitan. Cook until the seitan is nice and crisp all over, tossing now and then for even browning. Use a spatula to scrape the seitan into a small pile that will fit the bread.

11 Plop a few tablespoons each of caramelized onion and sauerkraut next to the seitan in the pan to warm up. When hot, layer the onions on the kraut, then layer the kraut on the seitan in the pan. Top with a slice of cheese. Add a splash of water to the pan, cover with a lid, and let sit until the cheese melts.

12 Lather up 2 slices of the toasted rye with Russian dressing. Using a spatula, place the pile of deliciousness on one slice of the bread. Spoon a bit more dressing on top and cover with another bread slice.

13 Grab some paper towels and stuff your face as you slowly fade into a food coma.

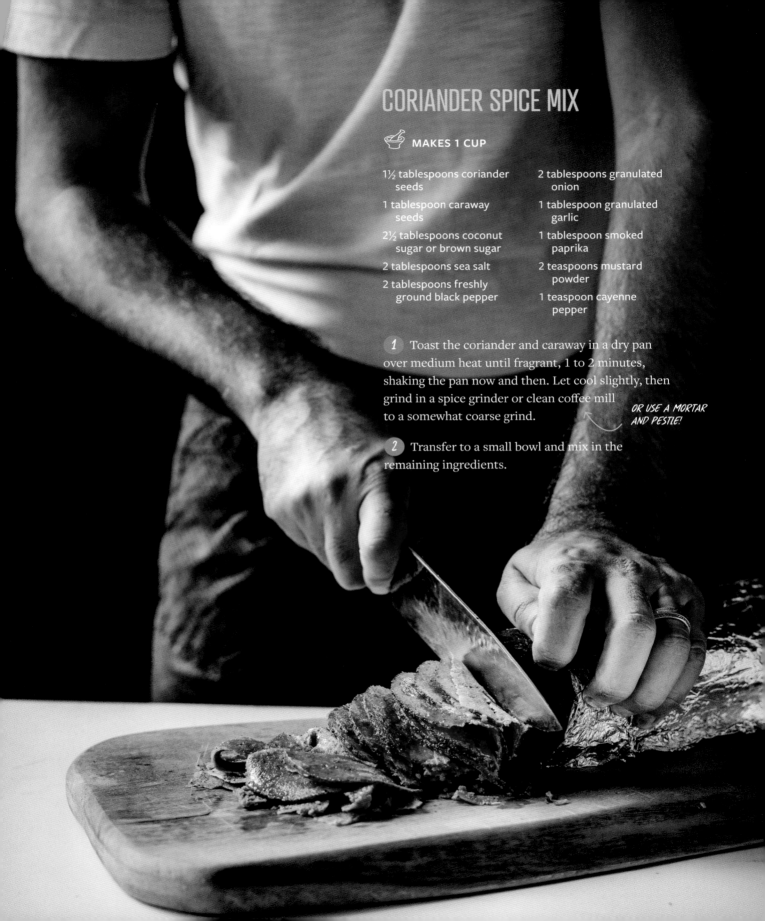

CORIANDER SPICE MIX

MAKES 1 CUP

1½ tablespoons coriander
seeds

1 tablespoon caraway
seeds

2½ tablespoons coconut
sugar or brown sugar

2 tablespoons sea salt

2 tablespoons freshly
ground black pepper

2 tablespoons granulated
onion

1 tablespoon granulated
garlic

1 tablespoon smoked
paprika

2 teaspoons mustard
powder

1 teaspoon cayenne
pepper

1 Toast the coriander and caraway in a dry pan
over medium heat until fragrant, 1 to 2 minutes,
shaking the pan now and then. Let cool slightly, then
grind in a spice grinder or clean coffee mill
to a somewhat coarse grind.

*OR USE A MORTAR
AND PESTLE!*

2 Transfer to a small bowl and mix in the
remaining ingredients.

GRILLED ALMOND BUTTER, CHOCOLATE, *and* RASPBERRY SANDWICH

Like a good ol' PB&J? You'll love this spin on the classic. Almond butter stands in for peanut butter, fresh raspberries brighten up the berry jam, and chocolate makes it all the more awesome. Plus the whole thing gets hot, melty, and crispy on the griddle.

 MAKES 2 SANDWICHES

4 slices whole-grain bread

3 tablespoons plant-based butter, softened

¼ cup almond butter

3 tablespoons berry jam, your favorite kind

½ cup fresh raspberries

1 tablespoon shaved or chopped dark chocolate

¼ teaspoon sea salt

A few mint leaves, torn by hand

1 Spread one side of each slice of bread with a small amount of butter, saving 1 tablespoon butter for the pan. Flip over the bread slices. Spread the almond butter on the unbuttered sides of 2 slices. Then spread the jam on the unbuttered sides of the other 2 slices. Top the almond butter with a layer of fresh berries, packing the berries in tight. Sprinkle the shaved chocolate, salt, and mint over the berries, then invert the jammy bread over the top.

2 Heat a heavy pan (such as cast iron) over medium heat. Add the reserved 1 tablespoon butter, swirling to coat the pan. (This extra bit of butter helps make sure the edges of each sandwich get crispy.) Put the sandwiches in the pan and cook until golden brown, 2 to 3 minutes per side, pressing just a little bit with a spatula to gently compress the sandwiches.

3 Slice on a diagonal and serve warm.

OPTION

- If you can't find fresh raspberries, use whatever fresh berries come into your market.

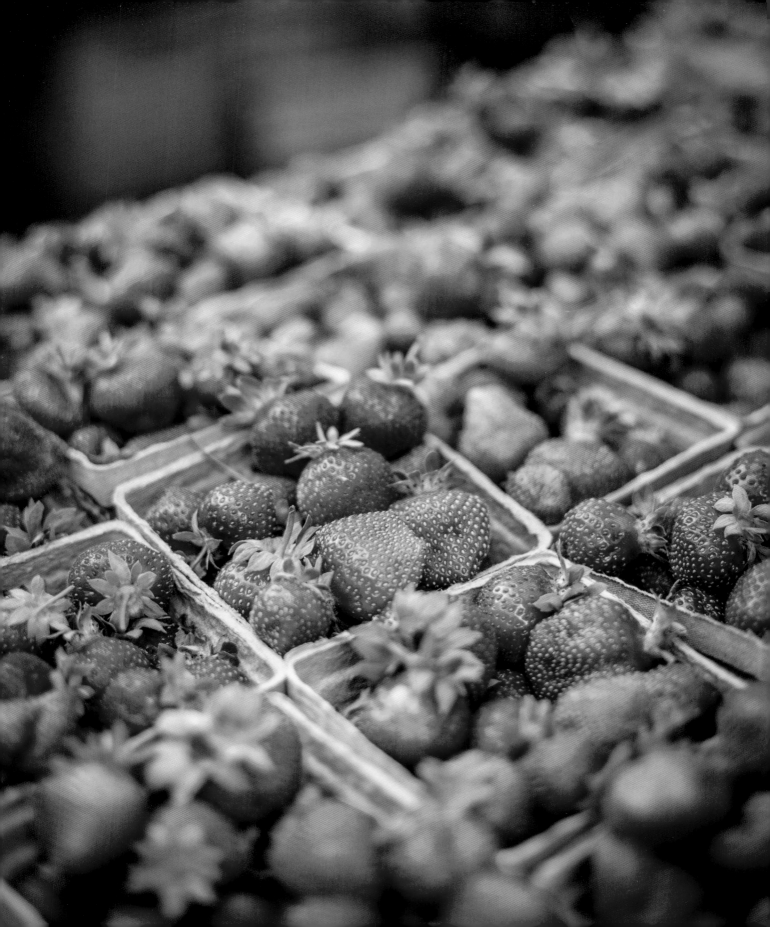

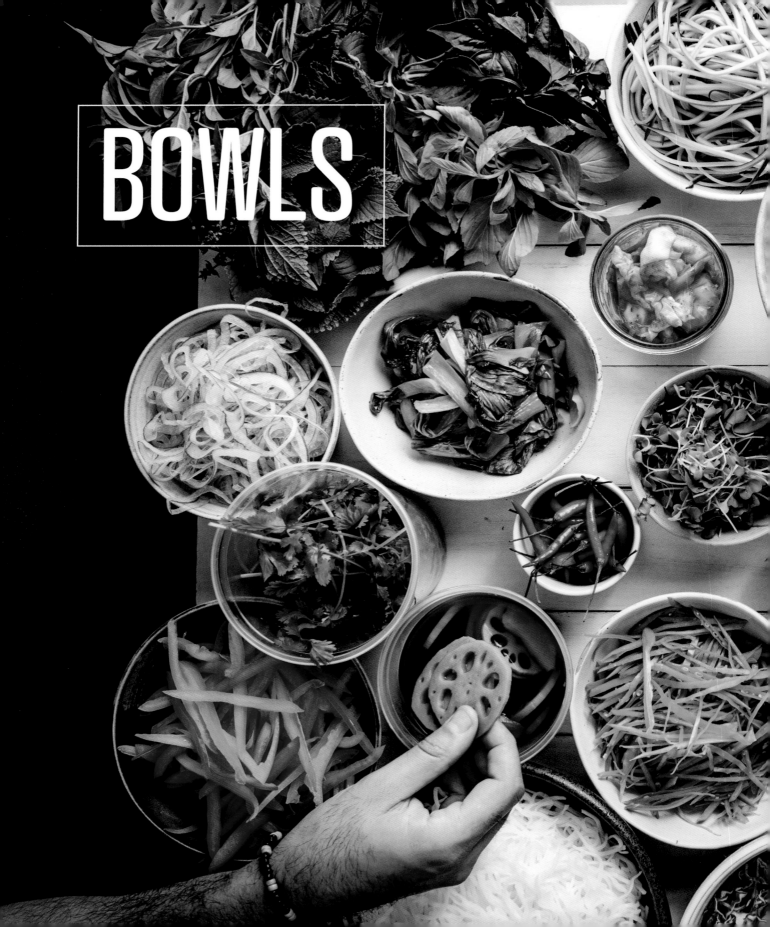

BOWLS

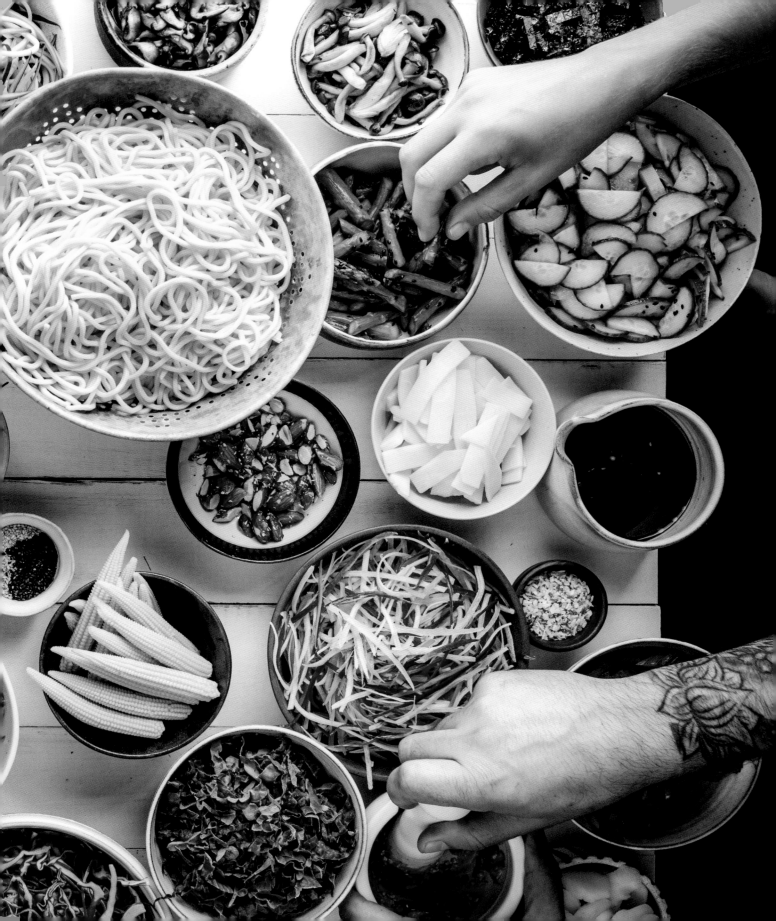

BUDDHA BOWL

u could have a noodle bowl every night and never exhaust the possibilities.
y out a table full of options and let your guests create their own signature bowl
ee whole Buddha bowl bar on page 138).

ODLES

ed vermicelli rice
noodles or buckwheat
noodles: cook al
dente (follow package
directions) and chill

ed lo mein, stir-fry,
or spaghetti wheat
noodles: cook al
dente (follow package
directions) and chill

cchini noodles

FOR THE RAW FOODIES!

UNCHY

ter lettuce: clean
and tear

rots: peel, julienne,
and rinse

l peppers: julienne
and rinse

ow peas: julienne

d onion: shave thin,
rinse under cold water,
and chill

thouse cucumber:
slice wicked thin into
half-moons; toss with
sesame oil, rice vinegar,
chile oil, sesame seeds,
mint leaves, and a pinch
of salt; chill

GRILL THE STALKS FOR MORE FLAVOR

Celery stalks: slice

Red cabbage: thinly shave

Kale: remove the ribs,
shred the leaves,
and rinse

Asparagus: steam; or
brush with toasted
sesame oil, salt, and
pepper and grill, pan-
sear, or roast at 400°F
for 1 minute; cut into
2-inch pieces on an
angle; chill

Baby bok choy: chop;
sauté in hot skillet
with 1 teaspoon
toasted sesame oil,
1 tablespoon sliced
garlic, and pinch each
of salt and pepper until
tender yet crunchy,
2 minutes; chill

Fresh steamed or canned
baby corn: rinse

Fresh poached or canned
sliced lotus root: rinse

Fresh steamed or canned
sliced bamboo shoots:
rinse

Canned sliced water
chestnuts: rinse

SHARP

Yellow onion: cut into
wedges with root end
intact; brush with
coconut milk and lime
juice and a pinch of salt;
grill and chill

Green onions: slice thin

Radishes: slice thin, rinse,
and chill

LOOK FOR DIFFERENT COLORS

TANGY

Lemon and/or lime:
cut into wedges for
squeezing

Pok Pok Som Chinese
celery drinking vinegar

AT 24VEGAN.COM!

FUNKY

Plant-based fish sauce

Local, wild mushrooms:
quickly pan-sear

HERBAGE

Cilantro, mint, parsley,
basil and/or Thai basil:
clean and pick leaves

SPICY

Homemade Badass
Sriracha (page 276)
or other sriracha

Red pepper flakes

Chile paste

Thai chiles: slice

SLICK AND SALTY

Ninja Tamari Glaze
(page 267)

Toasted sesame oil

Carrot Coconut Dressing
(page 272)

WHITE AND BLACK!

GARNISH

Sesame seeds

Crispy fried garlic or
shallots

Ninja Nuts (page 52) or
toasted almonds: chop

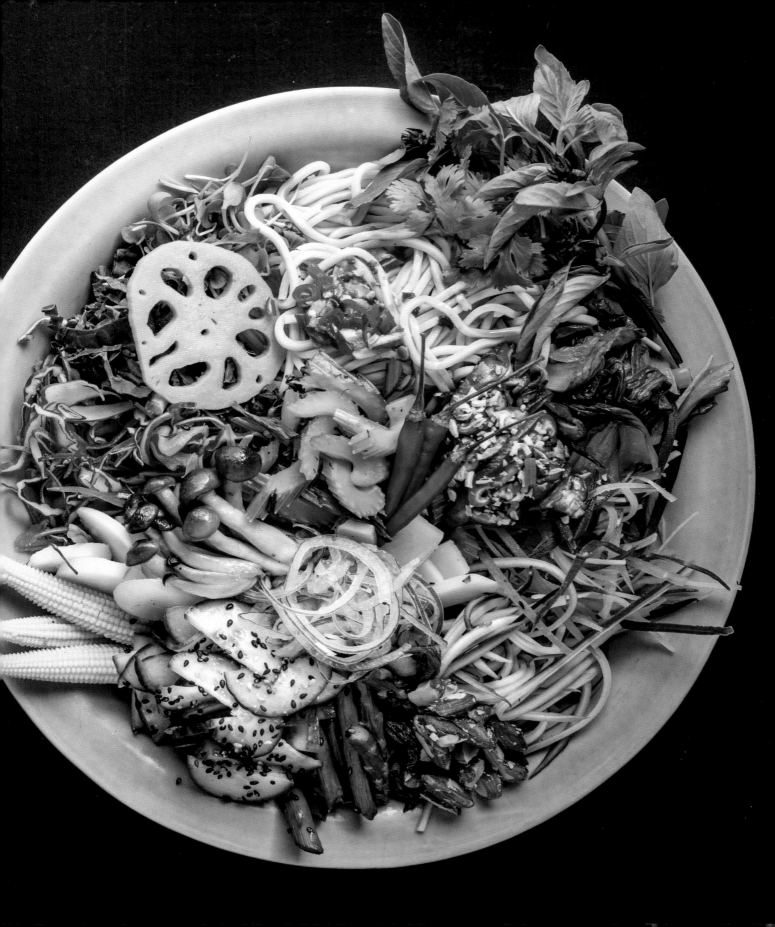

BANANA BLOSSOMS *with* COCONUT *and* CHILE

About fifteen years ago, I lived for a stint in the Philippines while revamping the menu for the Farm at San Benito, a health resort in the Batangas region. One of the chefs was from Thailand and usually made the staff meal. I fell hard for this dish. She made it with fresh coconut cream from the Farm, which tastes sooooo much better than canned. Use it if you can find it. The Filipino dish is called *ginataang puso ng saging*, which literally means "banana hearts cooked in coconut cream." Lime, cilantro, and chiles give this version a more Vietnamese spin. Either way, the banana hearts/blossoms are the star. They have a savory taste and chewy texture reminiscent of pulled pork. Look for fresh banana blossoms in an Asian market. Canned does not work well here. —*CHAD*

 SERVES 2 TO 4

1 banana blossom (about 1 pound)

½ lemon

Sea salt

1½ tablespoons everyday olive oil

3 shallots, sliced

4 cloves garlic, minced

1 tablespoon julienned fresh ginger

1 Thai chile, sliced into paper-thin rounds

1 can (15 ounces) coconut milk or coconut cream

2 tablespoons tamari or soy sauce

1 lime, halved

ASSEMBLY

3 to 4 cups cooked rice vermicelli noodles or rice

¼ English cucumber, cut into thin planks 2 inches long and ¼ inch wide

Shredded iceberg lettuce

Handful chopped fresh cilantro

2 green onions, minced

Thinly sliced Thai chiles, optional (if you like it spicy)

Lime wedges, for squeezing

1 **TO PREP THE BANANA BLOSSOM:** Rinse it well, and begin removing each layer of leaves, collecting the small banana blossoms within as you separate the leaves. Discard the tougher, outer layers of leaves. Continue removing leaves, retaining the tender inner leaves and small blossoms (image A).

2 Stack about 5 tender banana leaves at a time and cut the stack crosswise into long thin strips (image B). Fill a large bowl with water and a big squeeze of lemon. Drop the squeezed lemon half into the bowl. Place the strips in the lemon water (image C). I usually discard the small blossoms, but if you don't mind tedious work, remove the inedible stigma and small petal from each blossom as shown (image D). For very tiny blossoms, simply pinch off and discard the tips. When all the small blossoms are cleaned, chop them and add to the lemon water. Add about 2 tablespoons salt and massage the leaves and

RECIPE CONTINUES →

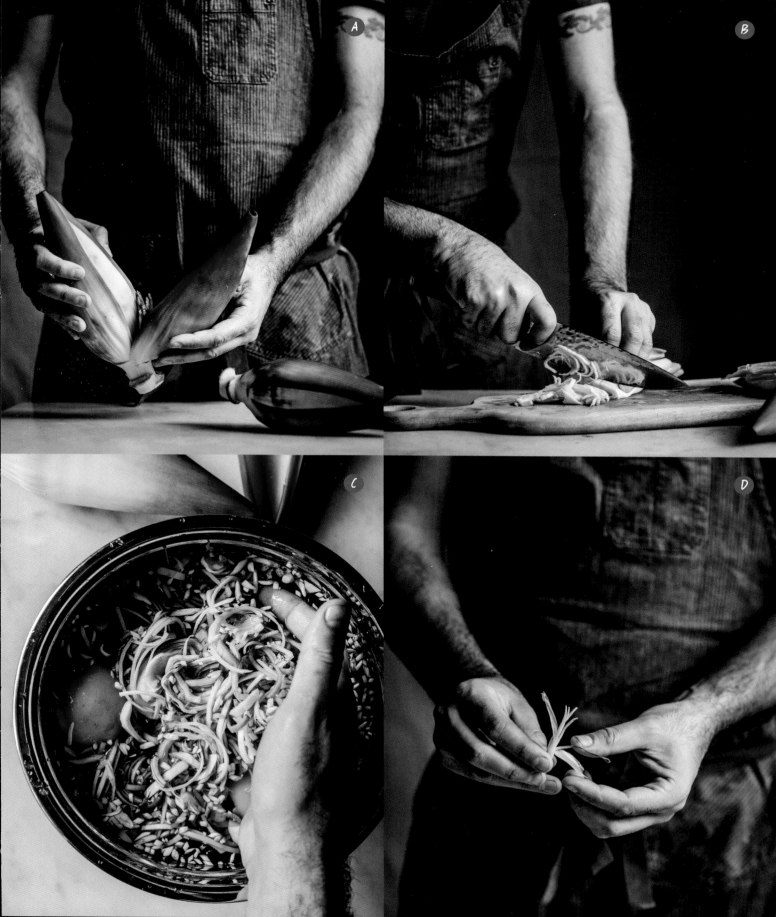

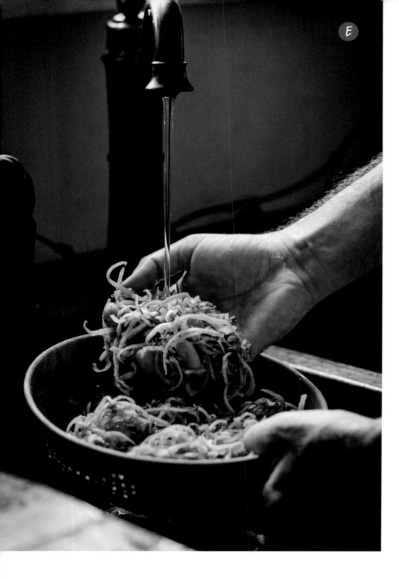

blossoms under the water, pressing them between your fingers for a few minutes. This process removes bitterness, and the water should become discolored. Drain off the water, then fill the bowl with fresh water, lemon juice, and salt. Repeat massaging and pressing under the water for a few minutes more. Drain off the water and pat the leaves and blossoms dry (image E). This unique ingredient is now ready to be cooked.

3 Heat a sauté pan over medium-high heat. Add the oil to evenly cover the bottom, then add the shallots and stir until they are translucent, 2 to 3 minutes. Add the garlic, ginger, chile, and prepped banana blossom. Shake the pan to spread evenly and sauté until the blossom takes on a bit of color and softens, 4 to 5 minutes, stirring to avoid burning the garlic.

4 Lower the heat to medium and stir in the coconut milk, tamari, and ½ teaspoon salt. Continue stirring until the coconut milk reduces slightly in volume. (Stirring helps keep the coconut milk from separating.) Remove from the heat and squeeze in the juice from one lime half. Taste and add more tamari, salt, and/or lime juice as needed.

5 _TO ASSEMBLE:_ Divide the noodles among 2 to 4 noodle bowls. Ladle in the coconut banana blossom mixture, and add cucumber, lettuce, cilantro, green onions, sliced chile (if using), and lime wedges for squeezing.

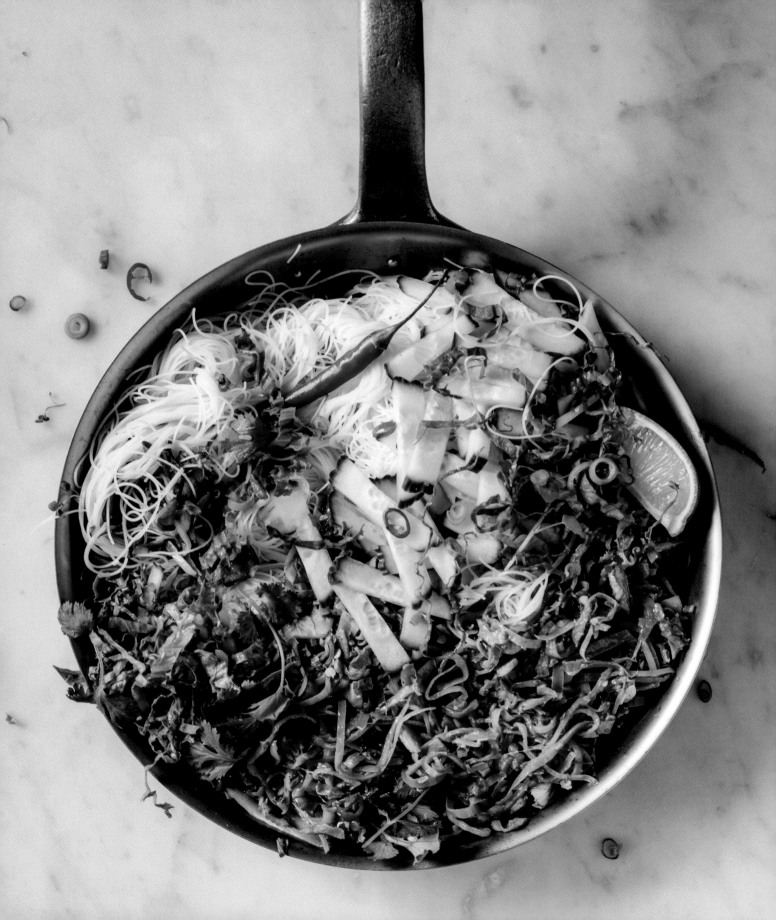

BIBIMBAP *with* BAMBOO RICE

Literally meaning "mixed rice," the Korean dish bibimbap is one of our favorite bowl foods. It's got so many different flavors, from the rice to the stir-fried vegetables (*kinpira*) to the tamari to the chiles. If you're adding tofu, make that first since it takes the longest. Everything else can be made while the rice cooks. Once you have all the components, the dish comes together pretty quickly. We like to use bamboo rice, a short-grain green rice infused with bamboo extract, because it's rich in health-boosting green chlorophyll. A glass of unfiltered rice wine makes a nice drink on the side.

 MAKES 4 BIG BOWLS

BAMBOO RICE

2 cups bamboo rice or other aromatic rice

4 cups water

1 teaspoon sea salt

KINPIRA

1½ tablespoons toasted sesame oil

3 pieces burdock root (see Pro Tip), peeled and cut into 2-inch matchsticks (about 1½ cups)

2 carrots, peeled and cut into 2-inch matchsticks (about 1½ cups)

¼ cup sake, or 2 tablespoons rice vinegar plus 2 tablespoons water

2 tablespoons organic cane sugar

1 teaspoon sea salt

BRAISED SHIITAKES

3 cups small shiitake mushrooms

2 tablespoons tamari or soy sauce

2 tablespoons sake, or 1½ tablespoons rice vinegar plus 1½ tablespoons water

1 tablespoon agave syrup

1 teaspoon minced fresh ginger

1 teaspoon sambal oelek or other chile paste, optional

2 tablespoons mild-tasting oil

KALE

1 bunch kale, ribs removed (4 cups leaves)

ASSEMBLY

4 cups Sesame Bean Sprouts (page 149)

1 cup cubed Baked Lemongrass Tofu (page 124), optional

1 teaspoon toasted sesame seeds, for garnish

3 nori sheets, cut into thin strips, for garnish

Thinly sliced red chiles, for garnish

Tamari or soy sauce, for serving

Homemade Badass Sriracha (page 276) or other sriracha, optional

1 *FOR THE RICE:* Combine the rice, water, and salt in a medium saucepan. Cover and bring to a boil over high heat. Cut the heat to low and simmer, covered, until the liquid is absorbed, 20 to 25 minutes. Remove from the heat and let steam with the lid on for 10 minutes. Fluff with a fork and set aside.

2 *FOR THE KINPIRA:* Heat a wok or heavy skillet over high heat. When wicked hot, swirl the sesame oil around the pan. Add the burdock and carrots, toss to coat with the oil, then quickly spread in a single layer in the pan. Cook, without stirring, until the vegetables brown lightly on the underside, about a minute. Add the sake, stirring to deglaze the browned bits from the bottom of the pan. Add the sugar and salt and toss to coat the vegetables. Remove from the heat. The vegetables should still have a crunchy texture.

3 **FOR THE SHIITAKES**: Remove the shiitake stems and reserve for another use (you can use them in the Mushroom Stock on page 284). In a small bowl or cup, make a sauce by whisking together the tamari, sake, agave, ginger, and sambal oelek (if using).

4 Wipe out the wok or heavy skillet, then heat over high heat. When hot, swirl the mild oil around the pan. Add the shiitake caps, toss to coat with oil, then spread in a single layer in the pan. Cook without stirring until the shiitakes brown lightly on the underside, about a minute. Pour the sauce over the shiitakes and stir well to coat completely. Cook until the sauce evaporates, 2 to 3 minutes, stirring once or twice.

5 **FOR THE KALE**: Bring a pan of water to a simmer over medium-high heat. Put the kale in a steam basket, put the basket over the simmering water, cover, and steam until just wilted, about 2 minutes.

6 **TO ASSEMBLE**: For each bowl of bibimbap, place a generous amount of rice in the center, then around it arrange small piles of kinpira, steamed kale, braised shiitakes, sesame bean sprouts, and cubed tofu (if using). Garnish with sesame seeds, nori strips, and chiles, and serve with tamari and badass sriracha (if you like) for drizzling.

> **Pro Tip**
> *Look for burdock root at an Asian market or Whole Foods Market. If you can't find it, use parsnips, kohlrabi, or even more carrots instead.*

RECIPE CONTINUES →

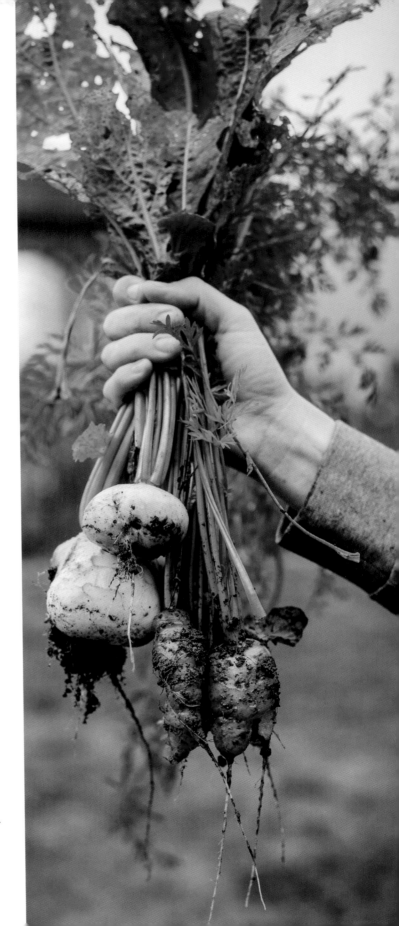

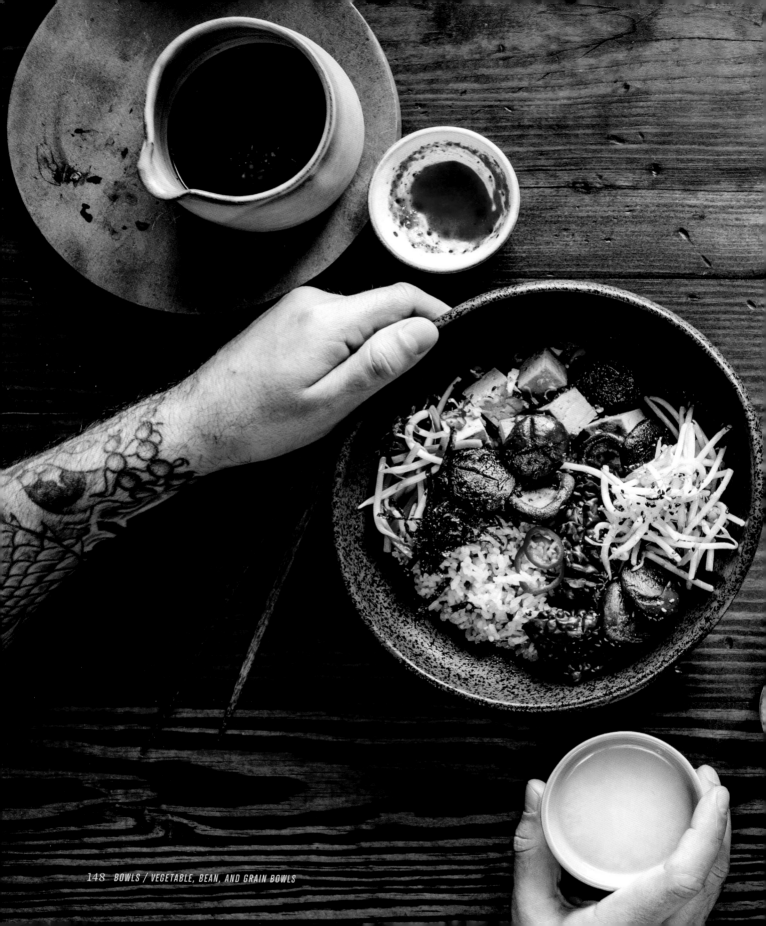

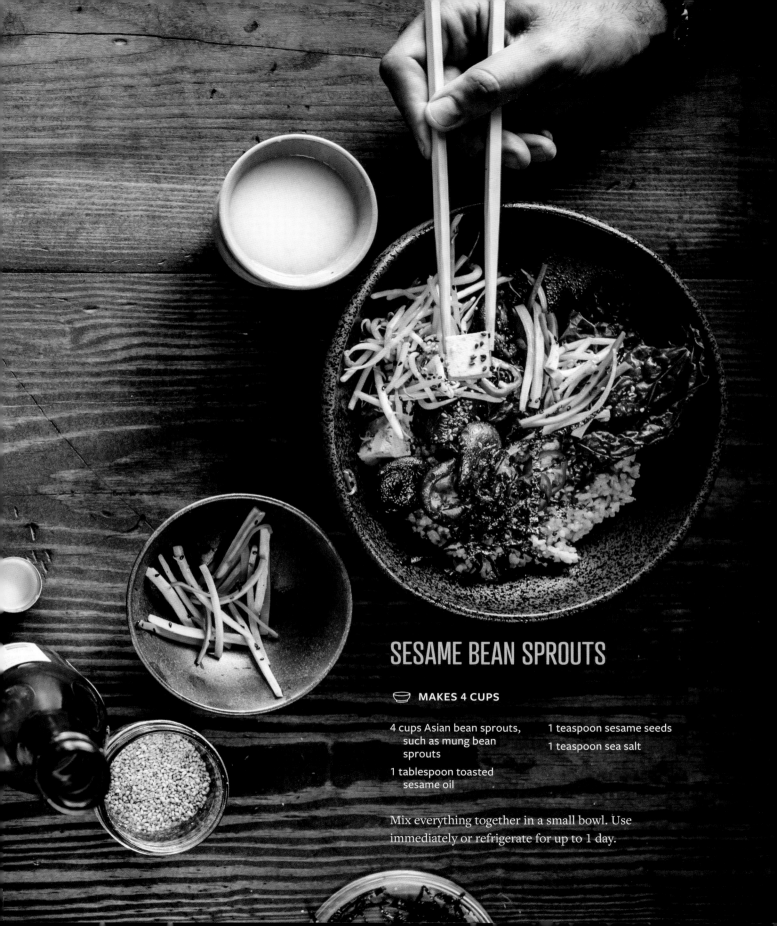

SESAME BEAN SPROUTS

🥣 **MAKES 4 CUPS**

4 cups Asian bean sprouts, such as mung bean sprouts

1 tablespoon toasted sesame oil

1 teaspoon sesame seeds

1 teaspoon sea salt

Mix everything together in a small bowl. Use immediately or refrigerate for up to 1 day.

SLOW-COOKED CORONA BEANS
with ROSEMARY *and* LOTS *of* GARLIC

Rancho Gordo grows some of our favorite heirloom beans. Their Corona beans have a meaty texture and a flavor closer to buttery than beany. Their thick skin can even crisp up in a hot pan. We love to cook these in a big cast-iron pot—sometimes over a wood fire when we're grilling other foods. If you can't find Coronas, go for gigantes, a similar heirloom bean. Either way, make a big batch. Serve some beans as a side dish or antipasto with a drizzle of good olive oil and some baguette. You can blend up the remaining beans with some stock or olive oil for an incredible "butter" to use as a dip, spread, or creamy sauce (see the Option). The Corona butter is what we serve with our King Oyster Scallops (page 79). —*CHAD*

 SERVES 6 TO 8 AS A SIDE DISH

1 pound dried Corona beans

About 8 cups Vegetable Stock (page 284) or store-bought low-sodium

8 cloves garlic, chopped coarse

3 to 4 sprigs fresh rosemary

2 bay leaves

2 dried red chiles, such as cayenne

½ teaspoon sea salt

½ teaspoon freshly ground black pepper

 1 Soak the beans overnight in water to cover.

2 Drain the beans and place in a large heavy pot or Dutch oven. Add the remaining ingredients and bring to a boil over high heat. Reduce the heat so the liquid simmers, cover, and simmer gently until the beans are tender, about 1 hour. Test by pressing one bean on a cutting board: It should crush easily but not be mushy. (While the beans are cooking, check the liquid level now and then; you may need to add a bit more stock or water to keep the beans covered during the entire cooking time.)

3 Serve hot with some of the cooking liquid.

OPTION

CORONA BEAN BUTTER: After cooking the beans, remove the rosemary, bay leaves, and chiles. Transfer half of the beans and their liquid to a bowl or stand blender, add ⅓ cup olive oil, and blend until very smooth. Use immediately or refrigerate for a few days, then spread anywhere just like butter. Makes about 2 cups.

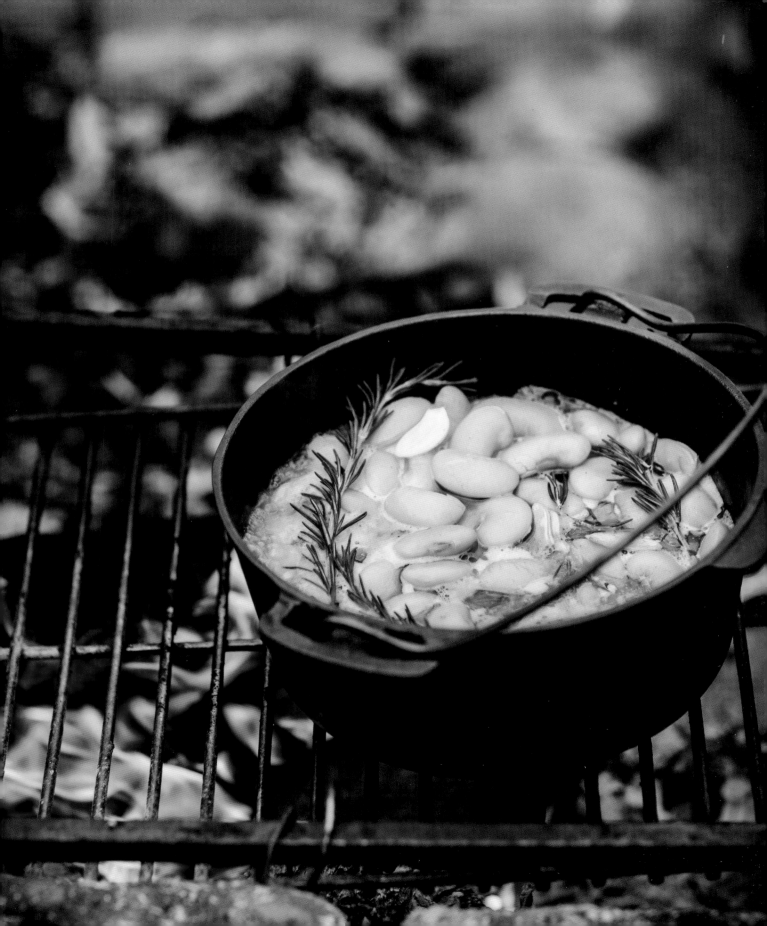

STIR-FRIED FARRO FAWCETT

JUST SHOWS YOU HOW WICKED OLD DEREK IS. —CHAD

Just saying the word *farro* reminds me of my high school sweetheart, Farrah Fawcett. That shot of her in the red bathing suit with her head back and a big smile...that pinup poster hung above my bed for many years. Making this dish puts a reminiscent smile on my face every time. It's basically a grain and vegetable stir-fry with grilled and charred veg for smoky flavor. You could just char the cabbage and celery by pan-searing them in a wicked hot wok or cast-iron pan. But I like to get outside to the grill. Feel free to use any seasonal veggies here. Keep the farro, though. It's one of the sexiest grains around. —DEREK

 SERVES 4 TO 6 AS A SIDE, OR 2 TO 3 AS A MAIN

1 cup farro, rinsed (see Pro Tip)

2 cups water

⅛ head red cabbage

2 stalks celery

3 tablespoons everyday olive oil

Sea salt and freshly ground black pepper

1 cup shiitake mushroom caps (stems removed)

½ cup diced onion

1 tablespoon minced garlic

1 teaspoon minced fresh ginger

½ cup cherry tomatoes, quartered

¼ cup Ninja Tamari Glaze (page 267)

1 to 2 tablespoons toasted sesame oil

1 tablespoon Pok Pok Som Chinese celery drinking vinegar

½ cup fresh cilantro leaves

¼ cup fresh flat-leaf parsley leaves

1 Combine the farro and water in a medium saucepan. Cover and bring to a boil over high heat. Cut the heat to low and simmer gently until the farro is tender, 30 to 40 minutes. Drain off any remaining liquid and set aside.

2 Light a grill to medium-high heat.

3 Lightly rub the cabbage and celery all over with 1 tablespoon of the olive oil, then season with salt and pepper. Grill the cabbage and celery, turning a few times, until grill-marked, 4 to 5 minutes total. Remove to a cutting board and chop the cabbage into bite-size pieces. Slice the celery stalks crosswise into half-moons. You should have about 1 cup each.

4 Slice the shiitake caps into strips. Have everything else ready to go because the stir-frying will happen wicked fast.

5 Heat a wok or large skillet over high heat. When hot, swirl in the remaining 2 tablespoons oil, then add the onion, garlic, and ginger and stir-fry for 1 minute. Add the mushrooms and grilled cabbage and celery and stir-fry for another minute or so. Add the farro, tomatoes, tamari glaze, sesame oil, vinegar, ½ teaspoon salt, and ½ teaspoon black pepper and stir-fry until hot, a minute or two.

6 Remove to a platter or plates and garnish with the fresh herbs.

OPTIONS

- You could use leftover grilled vegetables if you have some in the fridge.

- For more protein, scramble up some Follow Your Heart plant-based eggs or some cubed firm tofu in the wok. Remove to a plate before you add everything else. Then add the eggs or tofu back to the stir-fry at the very end.

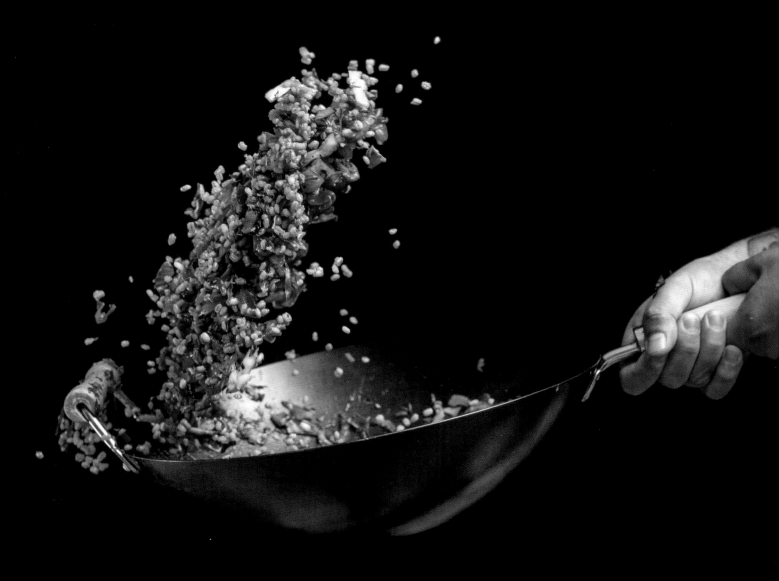

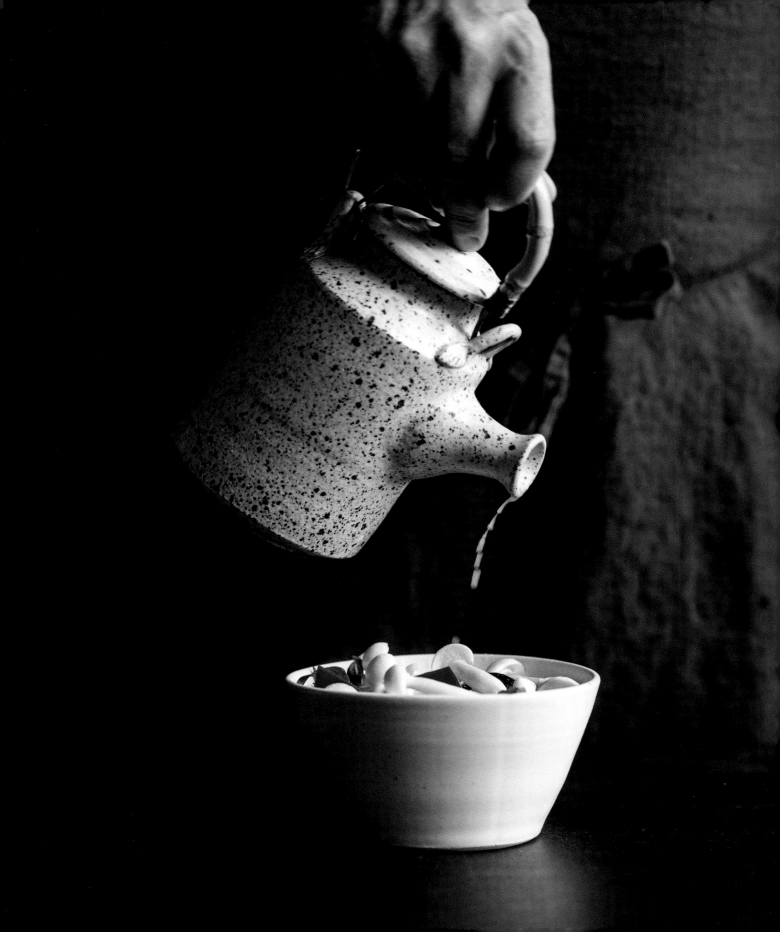

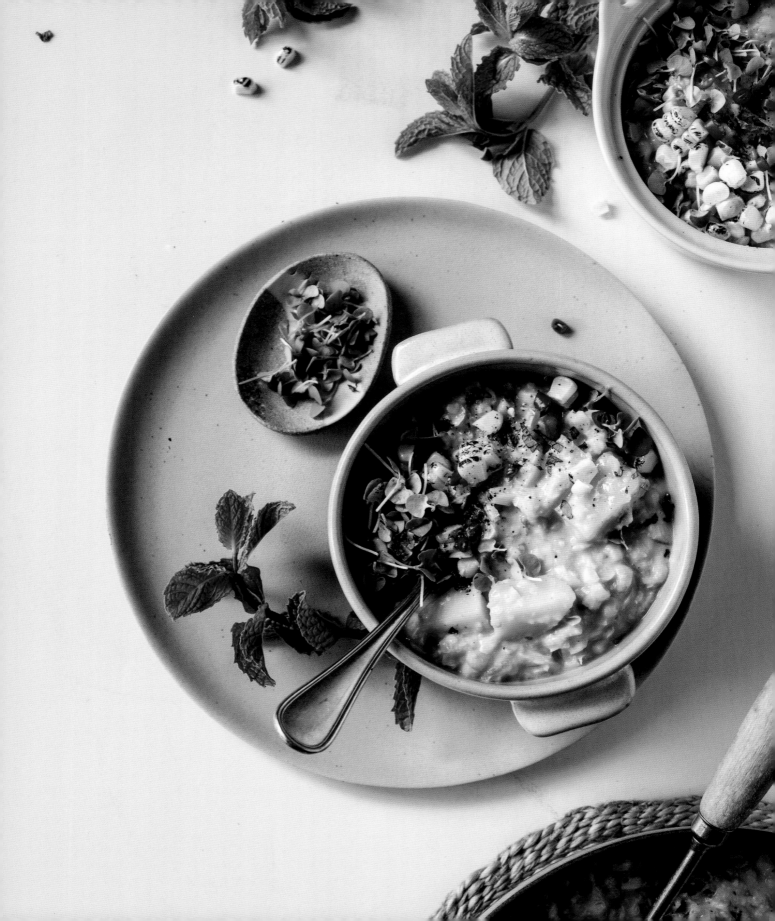

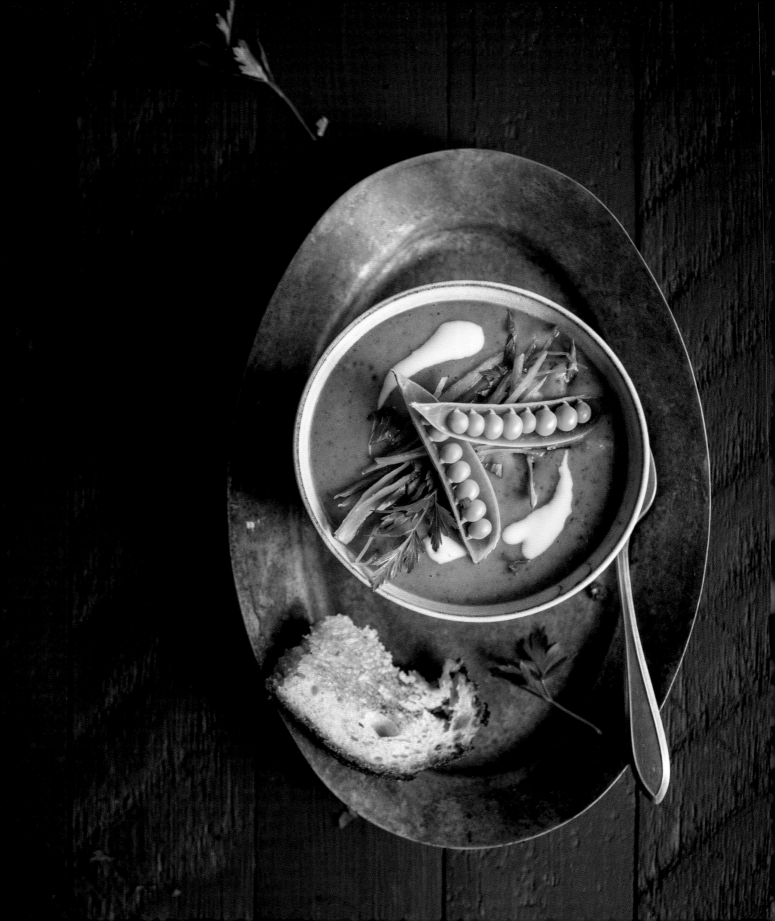

SPLIT PEA *and* CHARD SOUP

The U.S. Pacific Northwest grows some of the finest split peas, lentils, and garbanzos I've ever eaten. I keep the dried legumes in clear Mason jars in my pantry so I get inspired to cook and eat them often. I love me a good split pea soup, but I'm not crazy about the drab green color. So I blend in some fresh green chard at the end for a bright pop of green color and some extra plant-powered punch. Use this technique to brighten up any drab-looking green puree. P.S.: This soup is gluten-free and hearty as heck! —*DEREK*

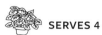 **SERVES 4**

1 cup split green peas, preferably non-GMO

6 cups Vegetable Stock (page 284)

1 cup diced Yukon gold potatoes, skin on is fine

½ cup diced onion

½ cup diced carrot

½ cup diced celery

7 cloves garlic, minced

1 bay leaf

1 teaspoon sea salt

1 teaspoon freshly ground black pepper

½ teaspoon granulated onion

2 large green chard leaves

1 Soak the split peas in water to cover overnight. Drain and place in a slow cooker (or see Pro Tip). Add everything else except the chard and cook on the low setting for 4 to 6 hours.

2 Rinse the chard leaves, then remove the leaves from the stems. (It's easiest to just cut along the length of both sides of the stem to remove the leaves.)

3 Remove the soup from the heat and discard the bay leaf. Add the chard leaves to the soup. Let cool until barely warm, at least 20 minutes, before blending. Then use an immersion blender or stand blender to blend in the chard real good and make the soup bright green. (If using a stand blender, remove the center lid to allow steam to escape and cover the hole with a folded paper towel.)

> **Pro Tip**
>
> *To make this soup on the stovetop, combine the soaked split peas and everything else except the chard in a large soup pot. Bring to a simmer over medium heat, then cut the heat to low and simmer gently for 2 to 3 hours, stirring often.*

OPTIONS

Garnishing ideas:

- Mexican chipotle sausage from Field Roast, crumbled and cooked
- Diced and roasted onions, carrots, and celery
- Fresh pea pods
- Cashew Sour Cream (page 77)

LOBSTAH MUSHROOM CHOWDAH

One spoonful of this stew and I'm transported right back to my New England home. The seafood-like texture and taste of lobster mushrooms is just mind-blowing. It's worth seeking them out. If you can't find lobster mushrooms, make the chowder with almost any white mushroom. The texture will be softer but the taste will still be good. —*DEREK*

🦆 🦞 **SERVES 4 TO 6**

3 russet potatoes, peeled and cut into 1-inch cubes

1 head cauliflower, cleaned and broken into florets

⅓ cup white miso

2 tablespoons plant-based butter, optional

1 large white onion, diced

3 stalks celery, sliced into ½-inch half-moons

5 cloves garlic, sliced

3 cups lobster mushrooms, cleaned and cut in 1-inch chunks

¼ cup dry sherry

1 tablespoon fresh lemon juice

1 teaspoon Old Bay seasoning

½ teaspoon smoked paprika

½ teaspoon sea salt

½ teaspoon ground white and/or black pepper

1 bay leaf

1 cup unsweetened soy milk

1. Put the potatoes in a medium saucepot and add water to cover. Cover and bring to a boil over high heat. Cut the heat to medium high, uncover, and boil gently until the potatoes are not quite tender, 8 to 10 minutes. Avoid overcooking the spuds; they should hold their shape and still be al dente.

2. Fish out the potatoes with a slotted spoon and set aside. Save the cooking water.

3. Measure the leftover potato water, add enough additional water to equal 7 cups, and return to the pot. Add the cauliflower and bring to a gentle boil over medium heat. Cook until the cauliflower is soft, about 10 minutes. Shut off the heat and let sit in the liquid for 15 minutes to let the flavors blend.

4. Transfer the cauliflower and cooking liquid, in batches if necessary, to a blender (preferably high-speed). Add the miso and adjust the center lid of the blender to avoid steam building up. Start blending on low speed, then work your way up to high, blending until super smooth, about 3 minutes total.

5. Heat a large soup pot over medium-high heat and add the buttah (which is optional; this soup can be made oil-free). When melted, add the onion, celery, garlic, and mushrooms and sauté until the onion is soft, about 3 minutes. If you skip the buttah, just keep the pan moving to keep the vegetables from sticking too much. Add the sherry and lemon juice and sauté another 2 to 3 minutes. Then mix in the Old Bay, paprika, salt, pepper, and bay leaf. Add the al dente potatoes and pour in the blended cauliflower mixture. Cut the heat to medium low so the soup is at a bare simmer. Stir in the soy milk and simmer for 30 minutes. Avoid boiling: Miso should never be boiled because boiling makes it lose its nourishing qualities.

6. Remove from the heat or keep on wicked low until ready to serve. Remove the bay leaf before serving and garnish at will.

OPTIONS

- Try roasting the cauliflower florets at 400°F for 30 to 40 minutes to add more complex flavors. Note that roasting will darken the color of the soup.

- To intensify the mushroom flavor, mix together the sherry and 1 tablespoon white miso and toss the 'shrooms in that mixture. Then roast the 'shrooms at 400°F for 25 minutes. When roasted, add them to the sautéing onions and celery as it says in step 5.

- *Garnishes:* Sprigs of cilantro or parsley, a dusting of Old Bay, and/or some oyster crackers

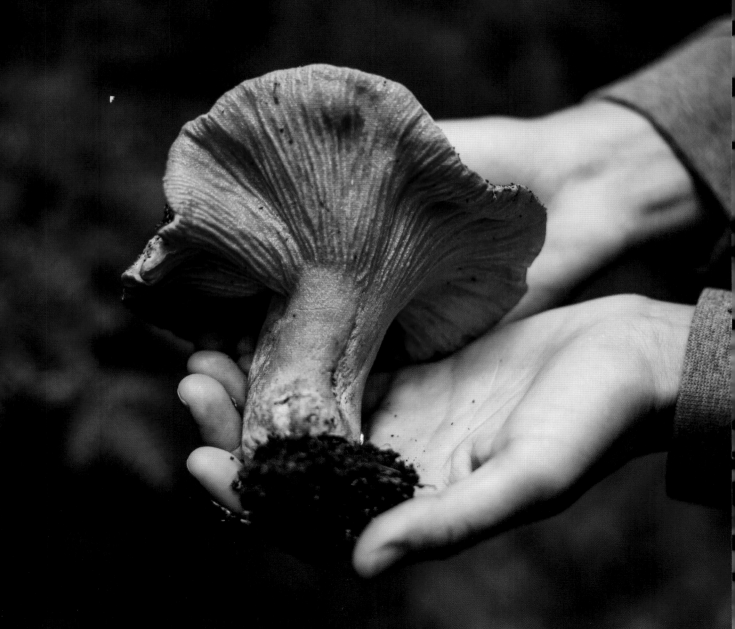

ROASTED CAULIFLOWER FAGIOLI

This is my riff on the classic Italian soup (pronounced *fah-ZHOOL*), usually made with beans and pasta. I replace the pasta with roasted cauliflower to push in some extra plants. It should be a pretty hearty, somewhat-thick soup, the kind you want to eat with garlic bread and a green salad. It tastes even better reheated the next day. Any carrots will work here. Purple carrots help deepen the color. —DEREK

 SERVES 3 OR 4, WHEN SERVED WITH SIDES

1 head cauliflower, rinsed

2 cups Nana Sarno's Red Sauce (page 265)

1 tablespoon everyday olive oil

1 cup diced onion

1 cup diced carrots

2 cloves garlic, minced

2 cups Vegetable Stock (page 284)

1 can (14 ounces) cannellini beans, rinsed and drained

½ tablespoon sea salt

1 teaspoon freshly ground black pepper

1 teaspoon granulated garlic

1 bay leaf

1 cup curly or dino kale, ribs removed, leaves rinsed and shredded

1 cup picked fresh flat-leaf parsley leaves, rough chopped

1 Preheat the oven to 375°F.

2 Cut the cauliflower into bite-size florets that your grandmother would eat. Put the florets in a mixing bowl and add 1 cup of the red sauce, tossing just to coat. Spread the florets on a rimmed baking sheet and roast for 30 minutes. The cauliflower should get somewhat soft and the sauce should glaze the florets with a few browned spots here and there.

3 Meanwhile, heat the oil in a large soup pot over medium heat. Add the onion, carrots, and garlic and sauté until the onion is translucent, 3 minutes. Add the remaining 1 cup red sauce and the stock, beans, salt, black pepper, granulated garlic, and bay leaf. Bring to a boil, then cut the heat to low and simmer until the flavors blend, about 15 minutes.

4 Add the kale and cook until wilted, another 5 minutes or so.

5 Stir the roasted cauliflower into the soup along with half of the parsley. Remove the bay leaf. Garnish with the remaining parsley.

OPTIONS

- For more heft, add ½ cup ditalini or elbow pasta after the soup comes to a boil. Return to a boil, then cut the heat to low and simmer until the pasta is tender. If the soup gets too thick, stir in a little water or red sauce.

- Sprinkle on some Follow Your Heart shredded Parmesan.

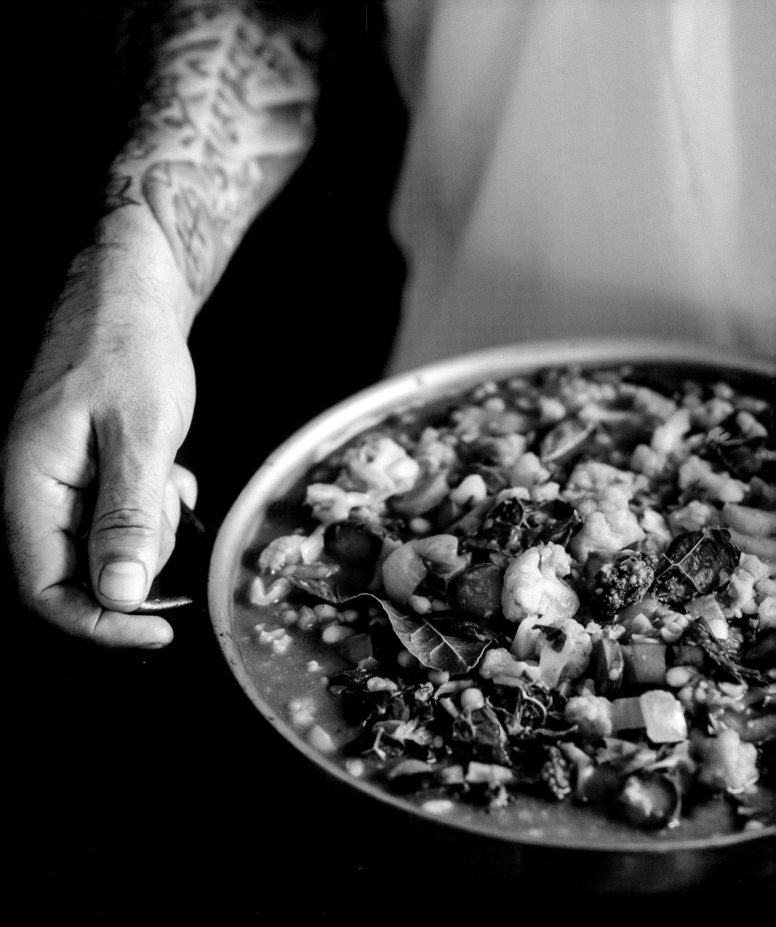

FOUR-BEAN *and* SWEET POTATO SLOW-COOKER CHILI

A good chili never goes out of season. We love this one anytime we want a rib-sticking stew made with foods we can feel good about. It has no added fat and couldn't be simpler to make: You just put everything in the slow cooker and let it cook all day. The recipe makes a big batch for a group—or for the week. If you have any leftovers (doubtful), freeze for up to a month, then reheat when you want a warm bowl of comfort.

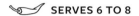 **SERVES 6 TO 8**

1 can (14 ounces) black beans, rinsed and drained

1 can (14 ounces) kidney beans, rinsed and drained

1 can (14 ounces) chickpeas, rinsed and drained

1 can (14 ounces) white beans, rinsed and drained

1 can (28 ounces) diced tomatoes, with juice

1 box (26 ounces) tomato puree

¼ cup molasses or brown rice syrup

2 good-size sweet potatoes, peeled and diced

1 large white onion, diced

1 bar (1½ ounces) hot chile dark chocolate, optional

2 tablespoons chili powder

2 tablespoons ground cumin

1 tablespoon freshly ground black pepper

1 teaspoon smoked paprika

1 teaspoon sea salt

1 jalapeño chile, sliced, for garnish

1 small red onion, diced, for garnish

1 cup picked fresh cilantro leaves, for garnish

1 Combine everything except the garnishes in a slow cooker (or see Pro Tip), and stir well to mix it all together. Cook on the high setting for 4 to 6 hours or the low setting for 6 to 8 hours.

2 Serve with jalapeño, onion, and cilantro garnishes.

> **Pro Tip**
> *To make this chili on the stovetop, combine everything except the garnishes in a Dutch oven and bring to a simmer over medium heat. Cut the heat to low and simmer for 3 to 4 hours, stirring now and then.*

OATMEAL BAR

Make a couple of types of hot oatmeal, set out some toppings, and invite your guests to breakfast. See page 168 for more options.

 SERVES 4

4 cups water

2 cups organic rolled oats

1 Bring the water to a boil in a medium saucepot. Stir in the oats. Cut the heat to medium low and simmer until the oats are tender, 5 to 10 minutes. Remove from the heat and cover until serving. If the oats thicken too much, stir in additional hot water.

OPTIONS

MULTI-GRAIN: Use a mixture of rolled oats, rolled spelt flakes, rolled wheat flakes, and rolled barley flakes. All of the grains cook in about the same amount of time and are widely available from Bob's Red Mill or your local market.

VANILLA SPICE OATMEAL: Add ½ split and scraped vanilla bean (or 1 teaspoon vanilla extract) and 1 teaspoon ground cinnamon along with the oats. Or use ground cardamom, nutmeg, ginger, cloves, or any combination of these warming spices.

CARAMELIZED APPLE TOPPING: Sauté ¼ cup diced green apple in 1 teaspoon plant-based butter over medium-high heat, stirring frequently, until browned and caramelized, 3 to 4 minutes.

POPPY SEED–CRUSTED ROASTED SWEET POTATO TOPPING: Preheat the oven to 400°F. Rub a small sweet potato with oil, place on a baking sheet, and put in the oven. Cut the oven heat to 300°F and slow roast until a skewer slides in and out of the potato easily, about 1½ hours. Cool completely (overnight if you want to make this the night before), then remove the peel. Roll the naked tater in poppy seeds (or chia or sesame seeds if you like) and a pinch of salt.

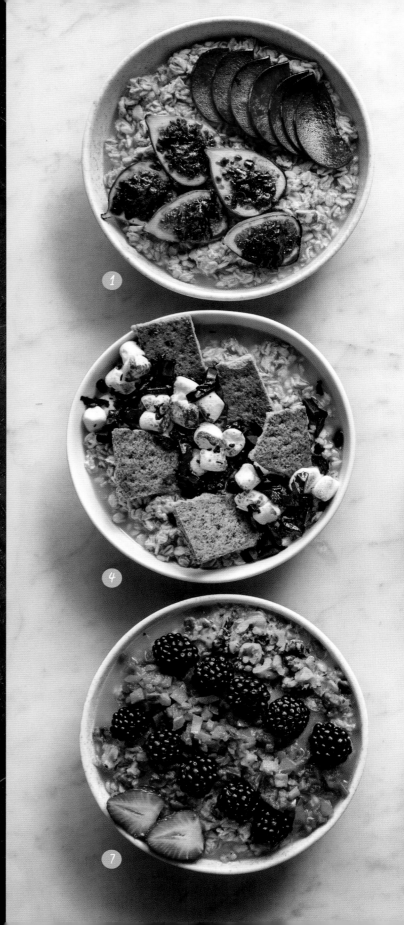

1. **VANILLA CLOVE FIG BRÛLÉE WITH PLUMS AND ALMOND MILK**

   SPRINKLE TURBINADO SUGAR ON SLICED FIGS AND BRÛLÉE WITH A KITCHEN TORCH

2. **DRY AGED GRAPES, TOASTED HAZELNUTS, AND BLACKBERRIES**

3. **VANILLA CINNAMON NUTMEG WITH POPPY SEED–CRUSTED ROASTED SWEET POTATO TOPPING (PAGE 167), RED JALAPEÑO, DRY AGED GRAPES, AND PECANS**

4. **VANILLA CINNAMON S'MORES**

   MELT THE 'MALLOWS AND CHOCOLATE WITH A KITCHEN TORCH!

5. **VANILLA NUTMEG WITH DRY AGED GRAPES, BRAN FLAKES, BANANA, AND BLUEBERRIES**

6. **VANILLA CARDAMOM WITH GRANOLA, RASPBERRIES, AND TOASTED PISTACHIOS**

7. **VANILLA SPICE WITH CARAMELIZED APPLE AND BERRIES (PAGE 167)**

8. **VANILLA GINGER WITH PEACHES, DATES, COCONUT, PECANS, AND MINT**

9. **VANILLA CINNAMON WITH NINJA NUTS (PAGE 52), BANANAS, BLUEBERRIES, AND MINT**

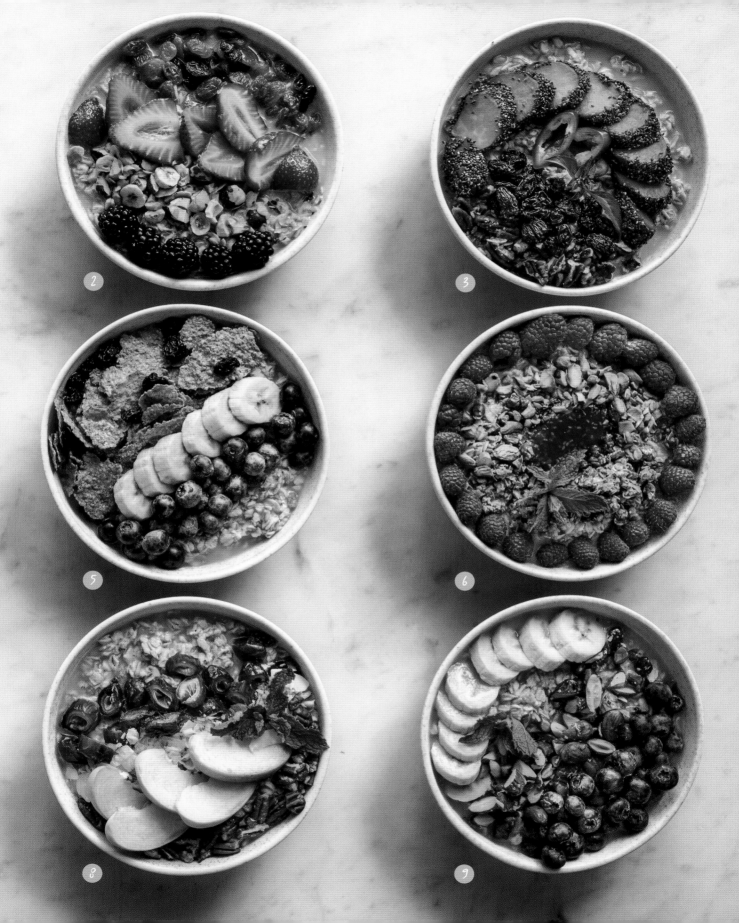

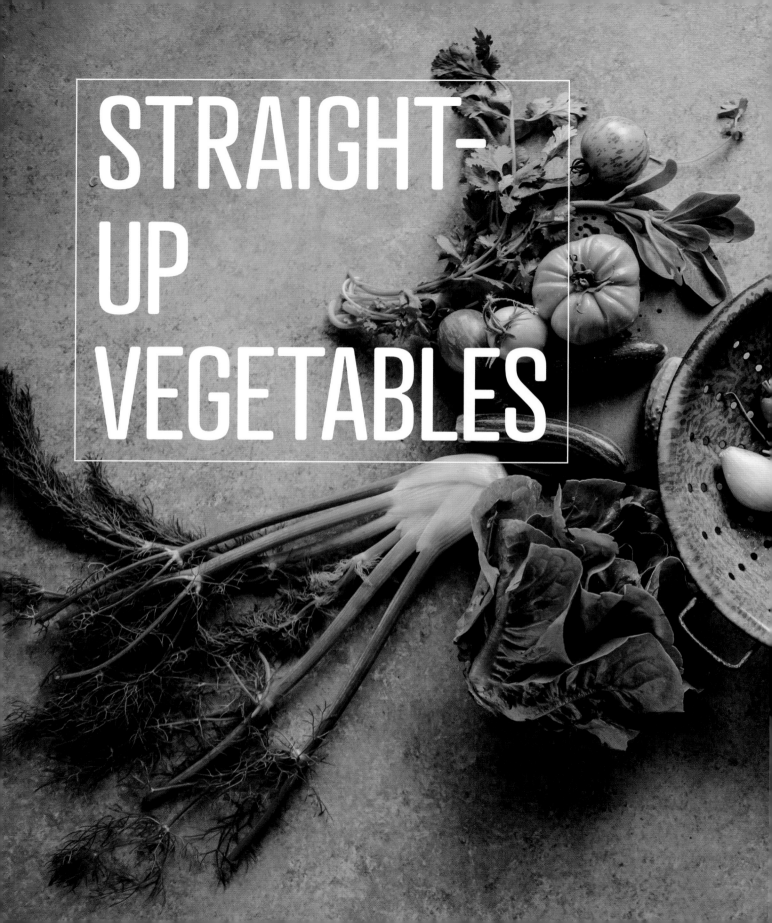

STRAIGHT-UP VEGETABLES

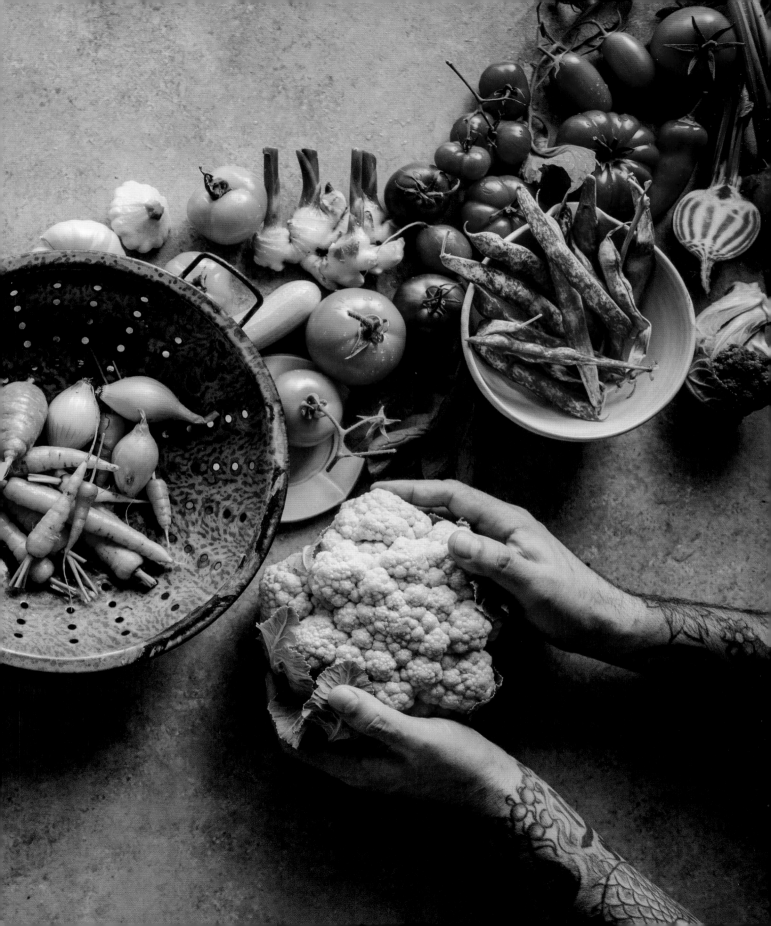

CAULIFLOWER RIBS

Cauliflower florets get the BBQ–sticky fingers treatment here. Look for a head of cauliflower that's not too tightly packed. You want to be able to break the whole thing down into larger individual florets with some stem on there. The middle of the cauliflower is sweet, tender, and perfect for this preparation. If the cauliflower has some leaves attached to it, leave them on. They get nice and crisp on the grill. Hope you like Korean barbecue: That's the flavor profile of the sauce that's slathered all over these sticky cauliflower ribs. Or check out the Options for other flavor variations. Eat these with your hands and keep the Wet-Naps nearby! —*DEREK*

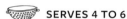 **SERVES 4 TO 6**

1 head (1 to 2 pounds) cauliflower

1 jar (12 ounces) hot pepper jelly (see Pro Tip)

¼ cup Ninja Tamari Glaze (page 267)

½ teaspoon sea salt

1 tablespoon sesame seeds, preferably a black and white combo, for garnish

¼ cup fresh cilantro or parsley leaves, for garnish

1 Light a grill to medium-high heat, about 375°F. For charcoal or wood, pile the coals to one side of the grill. For gas, heat only one side of the burners, and leave the other side off.

2 Begin breaking down the cauliflower carcass by holding the head upside down by the large center stem. Remove the florets from the center stem, leaving a long stem intact on each cauliflower floret. The stems should be reminiscent of ribs that you will hold as you gnaw the cauliflower from the stem. Try to make sure the rib pieces are thick enough and strong enough to stand up to saucing, grilling, and being eaten by hand when cooked.

3 Whisk together the pepper jelly and tamari glaze in a large mixing bowl. This is your sticky, sweet, spicy BBQ sauce. Wash your hands, add the cauliflower ribs to the bowl, and rub the sauce over the ribs like you're applying a generous amount of tanning oil to your bae. Coat all pieces thoroughly.

4 Scrape the grill clean, then place the cauliflower ribs on the hot grate. Grill for about 5 minutes per side. You're looking for good grill marks and a golden brown color with some burnt edges on the rib pieces. You also want the cauliflower to be cooked through yet still have some crunchability. If the ribs char before they're cooked through, move them to the unheated side of the grill, put down the lid, and cook gently until they are tender yet crunchy. If you have any leftover sauce, brush it over the ribs throughout the grilling.

5 Remove the ribs to a platter and shower with the salt, sesame seeds, and herbs. Eat with your hands.

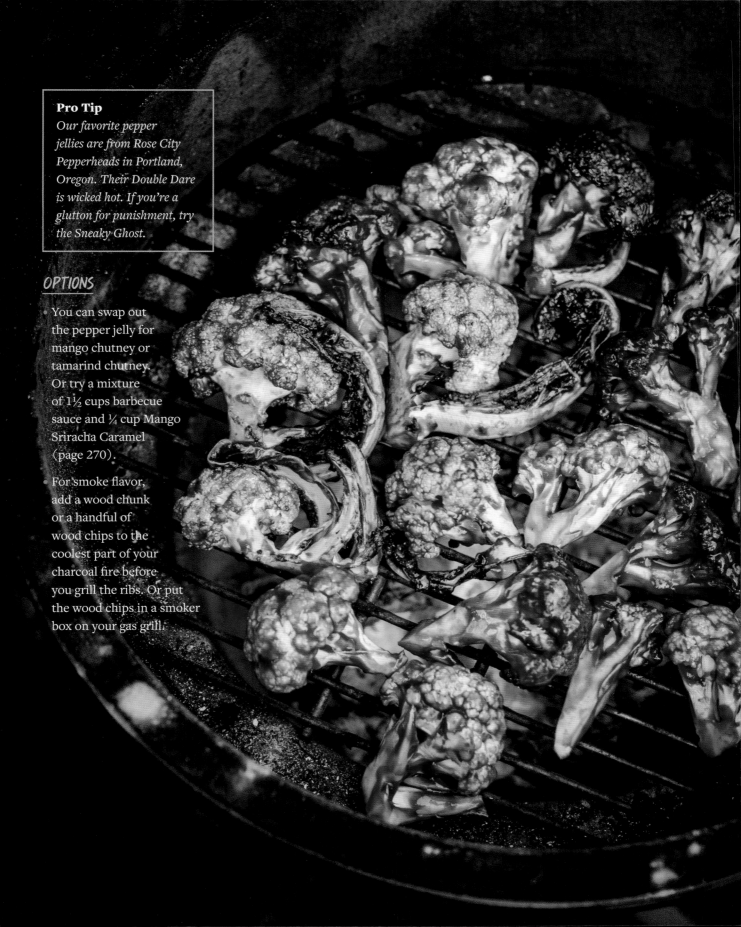

Pro Tip

Our favorite pepper jellies are from Rose City Pepperheads in Portland, Oregon. Their Double Dare is wicked hot. If you're a glutton for punishment, try the Sneaky Ghost.

OPTIONS

- You can swap out the pepper jelly for mango chutney or tamarind chutney. Or try a mixture of 1½ cups barbecue sauce and ¼ cup Mango Sriracha Caramel (page 270).

- For smoke flavor, add a wood chunk or a handful of wood chips to the coolest part of your charcoal fire before you grill the ribs. Or put the wood chips in a smoker box on your gas grill.

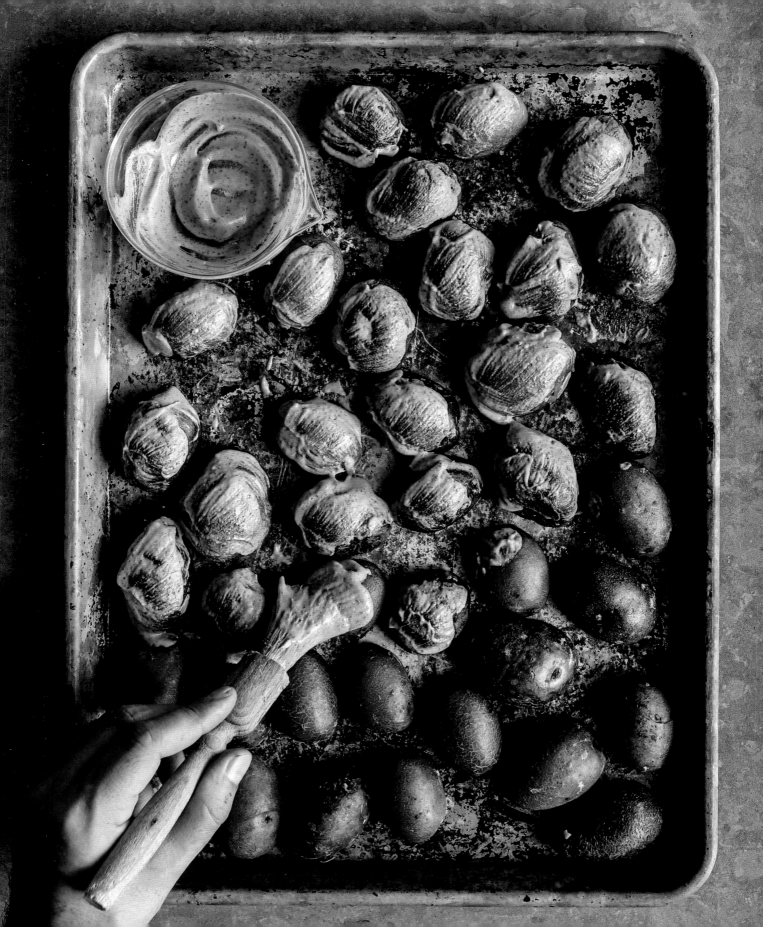

PAINTED DIJON POTATOES

Cooking is an art. One of the best ways to showcase that fact is to paint while you cook. Pick up a few small flat paint brushes from a hardware store. Then paint some sauce onto a plate before adding the rest of the food. Or paint a flavorful glaze onto vegetables. Here, we paint a yellow swath of Dijon mustard onto red-skinned potatoes. The rest of the seasonings hide secretly beneath the potatoes on the pan. Flavor and color—*voilà!*

 SERVES 4 TO 6

2 pounds red potatoes (see Pro Tip), unpeeled

¼ cup Earth Balance butter (at room temperature) or olive oil

4 cloves garlic, sliced thin into chips (about 1 tablespoon)

2 tablespoons chopped fresh rosemary, plus some sprigs for garnish

1 teaspoon sea salt

1 tablespoon freshly ground black pepper

½ cup Dijon mustard

1 Preheat the oven to 400°F. Scrub the potatoes, then cut each in half.

2 Smear the butter or oil all over a rimmed baking sheet. Arrange the garlic slices in a single layer over the butter. Sprinkle on half of the chopped rosemary, salt, and pepper.

3 Evenly arrange the potato halves cut-side down on the seasoned buttered pan, trying to completely cover the butter. Grab that paint brush and paint the red potato tops generously with all the mustard. Season with the remaining chopped rosemary, salt, and pepper.

4 Pop the pan in the oven and cut the heat to 350°F. Roast until the potatoes are tender and golden brown on the bottoms, about 30 minutes. You should be able to slide a fork in and out of a potato easily.

5 Arrange on a platter or plates and garnish with rosemary sprigs.

Pro Tip

Any smallish potato works great here, not just reds. Try little purple spuds, baby Yukon golds, or fingerlings. Just cut them in half lengthwise and lay them flat on the pan.

OPTION

- If you wanna get wicked crazy, paint the spuds with a mixture of half sriracha and half mustard instead of just the Dijon. Then drizzle on some Beet Blood (page 190). You could also swap in Mustard Seed Vinaigrette (page 271) for the plain ol' Dijon.

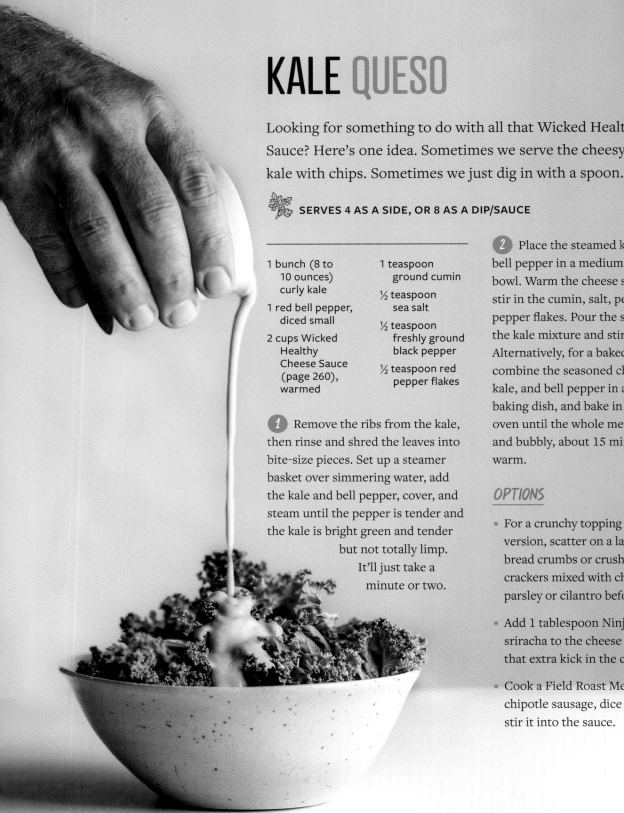

KALE QUESO

Looking for something to do with all that Wicked Healthy Cheese Sauce? Here's one idea. Sometimes we serve the cheesy steamed kale with chips. Sometimes we just dig in with a spoon.

SERVES 4 AS A SIDE, OR 8 AS A DIP/SAUCE

1 bunch (8 to 10 ounces) curly kale

1 red bell pepper, diced small

2 cups Wicked Healthy Cheese Sauce (page 260), warmed

1 teaspoon ground cumin

½ teaspoon sea salt

½ teaspoon freshly ground black pepper

½ teaspoon red pepper flakes

1 Remove the ribs from the kale, then rinse and shred the leaves into bite-size pieces. Set up a steamer basket over simmering water, add the kale and bell pepper, cover, and steam until the pepper is tender and the kale is bright green and tender but not totally limp. It'll just take a minute or two.

2 Place the steamed kale and bell pepper in a medium mixing bowl. Warm the cheese sauce and stir in the cumin, salt, pepper, and pepper flakes. Pour the sauce over the kale mixture and stir to coat. Alternatively, for a baked version, combine the seasoned cheese sauce, kale, and bell pepper in a 2-quart baking dish, and bake in a 350°F oven until the whole mess is hot and bubbly, about 15 minutes. Serve warm.

OPTIONS

- For a crunchy topping on the baked version, scatter on a layer of panko bread crumbs or crushed saltine crackers mixed with chopped parsley or cilantro before baking.

- Add 1 tablespoon Ninja Squirrel sriracha to the cheese sauce for that extra kick in the chops.

- Cook a Field Roast Mexican chipotle sausage, dice it up, and stir it into the sauce.

BROCCOLI *with* FERMENTED BLACK BEAN SAUCE

Beef and broccoli with black bean sauce was a favorite our mom made when we were growing up. For her stir-fry sauce, she used canned fermented black bean paste, which is made with soy sauce, sugar, fermented black bean puree, and sesame oil. I prefer whole fermented black beans, since they're easy to get now at Asian markets and have an amazing, earthy umami richness. Otherwise, this stir-fry is our ma's recipe exactly. The Asian holy trinity of ginger, garlic, and chiles—plus a little Shaoxing wine—rounds out the flavors. If you don't like broccoli, try green beans, asparagus, or bok choy. Add some mushrooms, edamame, or any kind of soy protein to make it a main dish. —*CHAD*

 SERVES 4 AS A SIDE DISH OR SMALL PLATE

BLACK BEAN SAUCE

3 tablespoons Shaoxing rice wine or dry sherry

2 tablespoons tamari or soy sauce

1 tablespoon agave or other sweetener

1 tablespoon sambal oelek, or thinly sliced fresh chiles

1 teaspoon toasted sesame oil

⅛ teaspoon ground white or black pepper

1 tablespoon cornstarch

VEGETABLES

3 tablespoons peanut oil

1 white onion, sliced thin

2½ tablespoons fermented black beans, rinsed

4 cloves garlic, minced

1-inch piece fresh ginger, minced (about 1 tablespoon)

3 dried red chiles, such as cayenne

3 cups broccoli florets

½ cup sliced water chestnuts (fresh or canned)

About ½ cup Vegetable Stock (page 284) or store-bought

1 **FOR THE SAUCE:** Whisk together the wine, tamari, agave, sambal oelek, sesame oil, and pepper. Whisk in the cornstarch. Set aside.

2 **FOR THE VEGETABLES:** Have everything prepped and ready to cook. The cooking will go really fast, so it's crucial to have everything prepped. Heat a wok or large heavy skillet over the highest heat. You want the pan blisteringly hot. Pour the oil around the edge of the pan to evenly cover the surface. Add the onion and stir-sizzle for 30 seconds. Add the black beans, garlic, ginger, and dried chiles; stir-sizzle another 30 seconds. Add the broccoli and water chestnuts. Use a spatula to press the broccoli against the wok to sear and get some color on it, 15 to 30 seconds more. Add ¼ cup of the stock and continue stir-frying to steam the broccoli and soften it, about another 15 seconds.

3 Add the sauce and stir-fry until the broccoli is crisp-tender, about 1 minute. The sauce should thicken and coat the broccoli. If it's too thick, add a little more stock so the sauce lightly glazes the vegetables. Remove from the heat and serve immediately.

GRILLED PURPLE CABBAGE
with MINT *and* PEANUT SAUCE

I love grilling cabbage. It cuts the bitterness and brings out the sweetness. The real star here, though, is the peanut sauce. It's creamy and savory with tropical flavors from ginger, lime, and coconut water. I love this sauce on almost any salad, but you could also use it to coat tofu or grilled vegetables, toss it with cooked noodles, or even drizzle it on savory oatmeal. —*DEREK*

 SERVES 6 TO 8

PEANUT SAUCE

1 cup smooth peanut butter

3 limes, juiced

⅓ cup tamari or soy sauce

2 tablespoons Ninja Squirrel sriracha

1 tablespoon chopped peeled fresh ginger

1 teaspoon chopped garlic

½ teaspoon smoked paprika

About 1 cup coconut water or water

¼ cup chopped fresh cilantro

CABBAGE

1 head red cabbage, rinsed

1 tablespoon toasted sesame oil

1 teaspoon granulated garlic

1 teaspoon sea salt

1 teaspoon freshly ground black pepper

A few fresh mint leaves, cut into thin shreds, for garnish

Sesame seeds, for garnish

1 FOR THE PEANUT SAUCE: Combine the peanut butter, lime juice, tamari, sriracha, ginger, chopped garlic, and paprika in a blender (preferably high-speed). Begin blending on low, then drizzle in just enough coconut water so the sauce blends and becomes pourable. Add the cilantro and blend just until incorporated. Use immediately or refrigerate in a sealed container for up to 3 days.

2 FOR THE CABBAGE: Heat a grill or grill pan to medium-high heat. Cut the cabbage lengthwise into eighths, leaving the stem on to hold the cabbage leaves together on each wedge. Each one should look like a plume of purple feathers. Put the wedges on a rimmed baking sheet and massage with the sesame oil. Season both cut sides of the wedges with the granulated garlic, salt, and pepper. Grill the wedges on all three sides until nicely charred, 5 to 8 minutes total. Charring gives the cabbage a lot of flavor.

3 Arrange the grilled wedges on a platter and drizzle on the peanut sauce like the artist you are. Garnish with the mint and sesame seeds.

Pro Tips

→ *You can use any coconut water (or even coconut milk) for the sauce. Harmless Harvest is one of our favorites. Add a teaspoon or two of toasted sesame oil too if you want.*

→ *To fill out the platter, add some grilled bok choy and tofu and a handful of bean sprouts.*

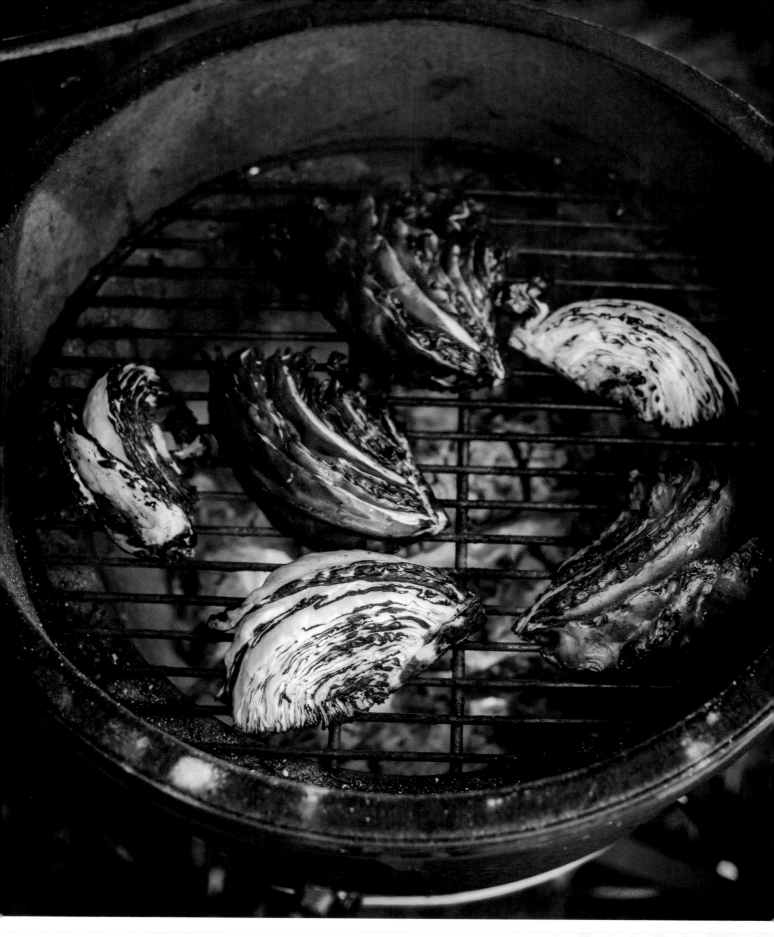

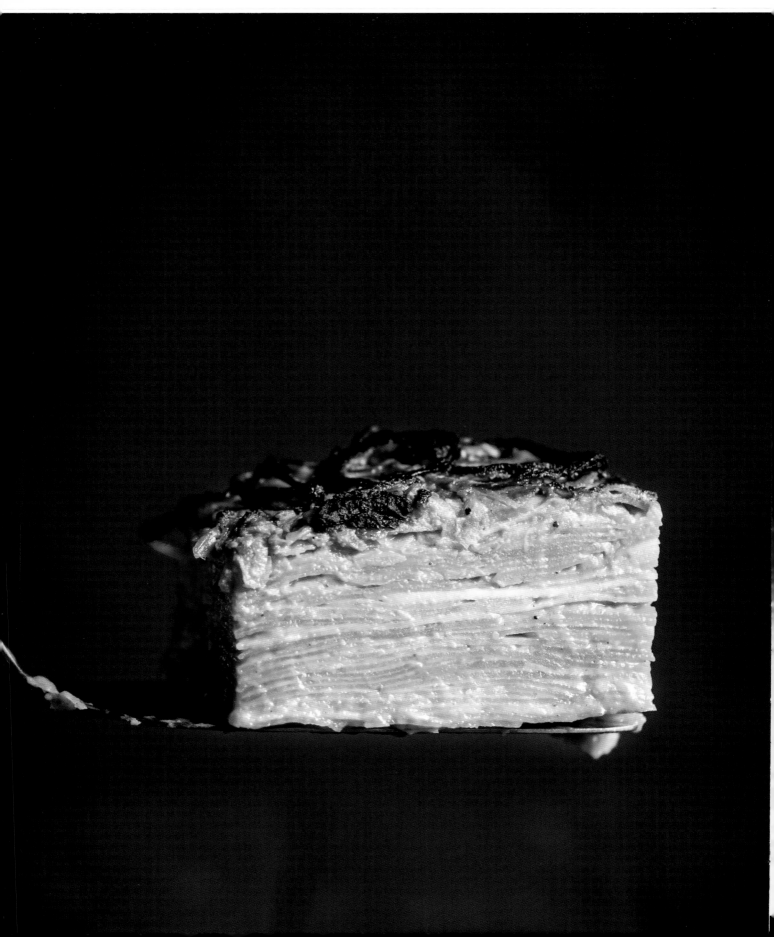

SWEET POTATO GRATIN *with* CRISPY ONIONS *and* ROSEMARY

Pssst...wanna be the hit of the holiday dinner party? Warm their hearts with this plate of deliciousness. Shhh...we don't have to tell them it's healthy and gluten-free, oil-free, dairy-free, and sugar-free. Just cut those yammers wicked thin and coat each slice with our Wicked Healthy Cheese Sauce. Layer 'em up carefully. Lovingly. Like you're tucking a child into bed. When you cut into the whole thing and see all those layers, it'll be like a work of art. Oh, how we love thee, sweet potatoes! —*DEREK*

 SERVES 6 TO 8

6 small sweet potatoes (2 pounds), peeled

4 red onions (1 pound), peeled and kept whole

Wicked Healthy Cheese Sauce (page 260)

1 tablespoon smoked paprika

1 tablespoon minced fresh thyme

1 tablespoon minced fresh rosemary, plus 2 sprigs for garnish

1 tablespoon sea salt

1 tablespoon freshly ground black pepper

1 teaspoon red pepper flakes

1 Preheat the oven to 350°F.

2 Use a mandoline to slice the sweet potatoes super thin. Mind your fingers! Slice the onions super thin on the mandoline. Rinse and set aside to drain.

3 Mix the sauce in a large bowl with the paprika, thyme, rosemary, salt, black pepper, and pepper flakes.

4 Add the sweet potatoes to the sauce and toss so each slice is well coated. Assemble the potatoes evenly in a deep 4-quart baking dish, layering the slices to make the gratin about 3 inches thick. Make it pretty. Pour just enough of the remaining sauce to thinly cover the top of the sweet potatoes.

5 Mix the onion slivers with that last bit of sauce and spread evenly on top of the sweet potatoes. Cover tightly with foil, trying to keep the foil from touching the onion and sweet potatoes.

6 Bake until the sweet potatoes are tender enough for a wooden skewer to slide in and out easily, 50 to 60 minutes.

7 Uncover and roast another 10 minutes to brown the onion top. Remove from the heat and let rest 10 minutes before slicing. Garnish with a couple of sprigs of fresh rosemary.

> **Pro Tip**
> *If you can swing it, make this dish a day ahead or the night before. Like lasagna, it sets and slices better and the flavors blend so it tastes even better when reheated the next day.*

SMOKY CHEESY ROASTED CAULIFLOWER HEAD

There's something primal about roasting a whole head of anything. This deeply browned whole head of cauliflower makes an incredible presentation and great centerpiece. I like to cook it to the point where the cauliflower meat is almost falling off the bone...I mean, er, the *stem*. Sometimes I serve it with barbecued foods to enhance the whole eat-with-your-hands vibe as you rip the cauliflower florets from the head. A side of Mango Sriracha Caramel (page 270) is perfect for dunking. —*DEREK*

 SERVES 4

Mild-tasting oil, for coating the pan

1 whole head cauliflower, rinsed

2 cups Wicked Healthy Cheese Sauce (page 260)

2 teaspoons picked fresh thyme leaves, plus some sprigs for garnish

1 teaspoon smoked paprika

1 teaspoon red pepper flakes

1 teaspoon sea salt

1 teaspoon freshly ground black pepper

1 Preheat the oven to 350°F. Lightly oil a baking pan that'll just fit the whole head of cauliflower.

2 Trim the cauliflower brainstem only enough so the head will stand upright. Leave any light green leaves on the head if possible. (The leaves curl up and get crispy in the oven, giving the whole thing a more rustic look. And they're totally edible.)

NOTHING WASTED!

3 Whisk together the cheese sauce, thyme, paprika, pepper flakes, salt, and black pepper in a medium bowl. Dip the whole head in the sauce and bathe the florets all over with a spoon, making sure it's completely covered and some sauce seeps into the inner catacombs.

4 Put the head, florets up, on the prepared pan. Save any extra sauce for basting. Roast the head until soft throughout, about 1½ hours. When it's done, a skewer, fork, or toothpick should easily pierce even the toughest center part of the head. While it's roasting, spoon some sauce over the head every 15 minutes or so to get it good and glazed all over. Let cool 5 to 10 minutes. No touchy!

5 When it's cooled down a bit (don't worry, it'll still be plenty warm), serve that bad boy whole on a platter and eat it with your hands. Or, if you're in polite company, slice into quarters and serve with the requisite tableware. Garnish with a few fresh thyme sprigs.

Pro Tip

Your best bet is to buy farmers' market cauliflower because the florets are usually a bit looser and the sauce can drip deep down into the caverns. If you get a really tight head of cauliflower, open up the florets a little with your hands so the sauce drips inside.

• For queso-style cauliflower with Texan flavors, use oregano instead of thyme and add 1 teaspoon chili powder and ½ teaspoon ground cumin to the sauce. Add 3 to 4 tablespoons Ninja Squirrel sriracha or some chile paste for even more punch.

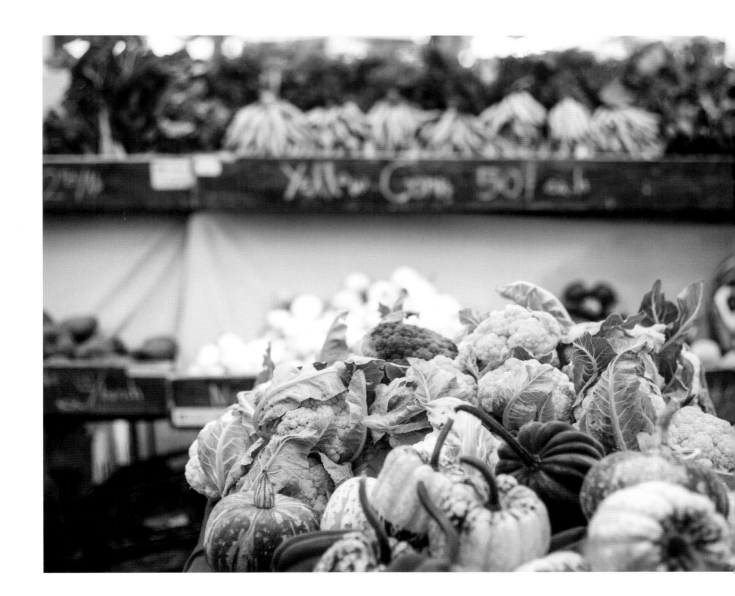

GRILLED EGGPLANT TENDERLOINS *with* BEET BLOOD *and* NINJA NUTS

Fire up the grill for this baby. A little applewood smoke throws it over the top. The beet "blood" is just beet juice boiled down with sugar and salt to make a deep red, sweet, salty sauce that adds complexity to anything it's spilled onto—like grilled eggplant. This bloody delicious mess makes a great family-style platter that hits all corners of your taste buds.

 SERVES 4

1 teaspoon toasted sesame oil

4 Chinese or other long, skinny eggplants, each 12 inches long (about 1¼ pounds total)

½ teaspoon sea salt

½ teaspoon freshly ground black pepper

Handful of applewood chunks or chips

2 tablespoons Kite Hill plain yogurt or other nondairy yogurt

2 tablespoons Beet Blood (page 190)

¼ cup chopped Ninja Nuts (page 52)

1 to 2 skinny red Thai chiles, sliced thin; or some chile flakes

Sprigs of fresh mint, basil, and/or cilantro, for garnish

1 Fire up your grill (preferably charcoal) to medium-high heat, about 450°F.

2 Pour the sesame oil into your palms and rub it between your hands like a massage therapist. Now, rub those eggplants all over until they're nice and happy. Season all over with the salt and pepper.

3 When the fire is ready, toss the applewood chunks or chips onto the coolest part of the fire so they slowly smolder instead of incinerating. When you see lots of smoke, put the eggplants on the grill directly over the heat and close the lid. Cook, turning every few minutes, until the purple color on the skin fades a bit and the eggplants shrink slightly, 6 to 10 minutes total. These cook up pretty quickly. The eggplant should become soft and easy to pierce with a skewer.

4 Remove to a cutting board and let sit a minute or two before carving. Slice on a diagonal into ovals about 1 inch thick. Arrange on a platter and begin your art project.

5 First drizzle on a little yogurt, then the beet blood. Adorn with the nuts and sliced chiles, then garnish with the herbs.

OPTIONS

- To roast the eggplants instead of grilling them, preheat the oven to 400°F. Roast on a baking sheet until soft enough to pierce easily with a skewer, 20 to 30 minutes. You won't get the smokiness of the grill, but all the other flavors will pop.

- For some spicy-sweet razzle dazzle, drizzle on about 1 tablespoon Mango Sriracha Caramel (page 270) along with the beet blood. Or just go sweet and drizzle on a little agave or maple syrup.

RECIPE CONTINUES →

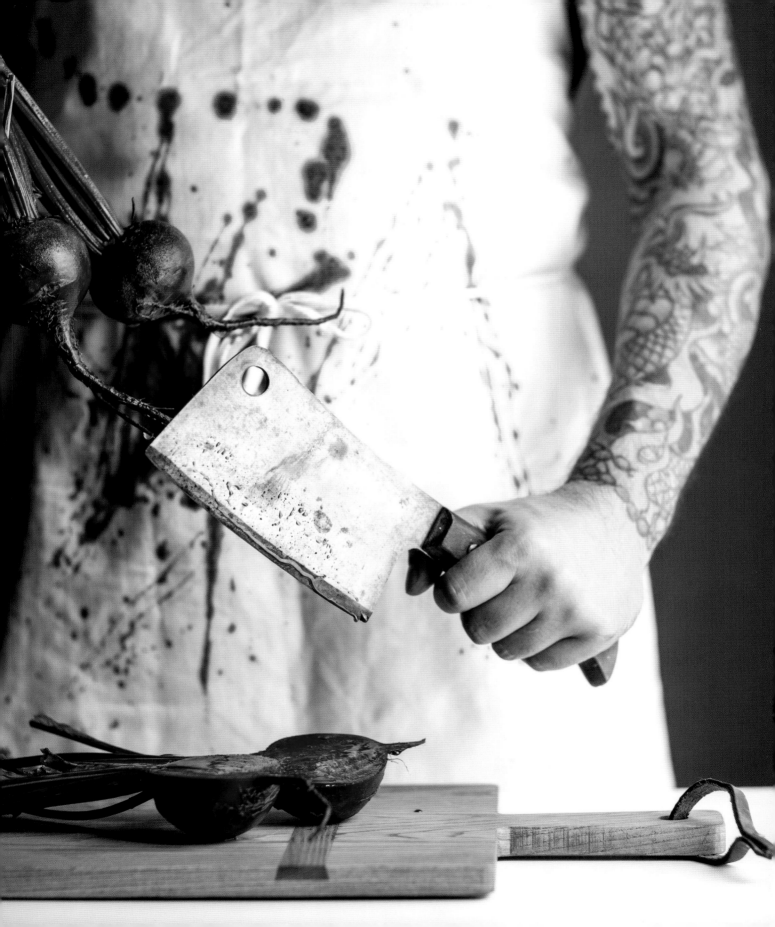

BEET BLOOD

 MAKES ABOUT 1¼ CUPS

2 cups (16 ounces) beet
   juice (see Pro Tip)

1½ cups organic cane
   sugar

1 teaspoon sea salt

1 Whisk everything together in a small saucepot. Bring to a slow simmering boil over medium heat, stirring occasionally with a wooden spoon. Let the mixture simmer and reduce in volume by about half, 30 minutes or so. The consistency should be like thin syrup or warm maple syrup. When it cools, it will get thicker, but for now, shoot for thin syrup, testing the consistency with the wooden spoon. But don't taste it—it's as hot as molten lava at this point!

2 When it's the consistency of thin syrup, remove the pot from the heat and let the syrup cool just until warm but still pourable, 5 to 10 minutes. Pour it into a glass jar and screw on the lid. Refrigerate for up to 1 month. When cold, the consistency will be thicker, somewhere between maple syrup and honey. Bring to room temperature or slightly warm it before serving.

Pro Tip

To get 2 cups of beet juice, run about 2½ pounds of beets (8 to 10 medium) through a juicer— greens and everything. Or pick up some beet juice at a local juice bar or natural foods store.

OPTION

BEET BLOOD WITH MERLOT: To switch up the flavor, replace half of the beet juice with a jammy New World merlot.

SUMMER VEGETABLE CARPACCIO

This isn't a recipe! It's a showcase for whatever vegetables are at the peak of ripeness near you this summer. Go for the freshest veg you can get. Arrange thin slices on a board or platter (have fun alternating colors and shapes!), then scatter on some wicked good olive oil, crunchy salt, and picked herb leaves and add a squeeze of lemon.

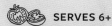 **SERVES 6+**

- Your favorite in-season vegetables, such as heirloom tomatoes, radishes, zucchini, crookneck squash, fennel, beets, or kohlrabi, sliced paper-thin using a mandoline

- Toasted pine nuts

- Fresh-picked tender herb leaves—especially basil, mint, parsley, tarragon, and/or dill

- Shallots, garlic, and/or chiles sliced paper-thin—go easy on these

- Your best-quality extra-virgin olive oil

- Meyer lemon, squeezed

- Flake salt, such as Maldon

- Freshly cracked black pepper

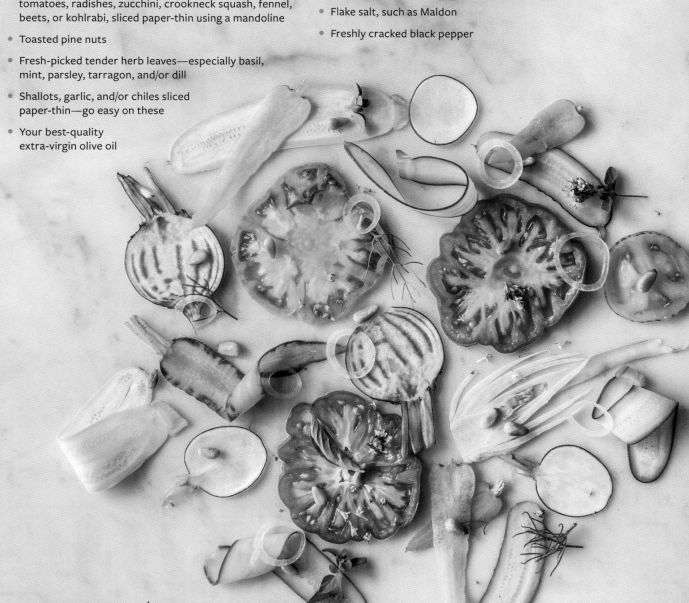

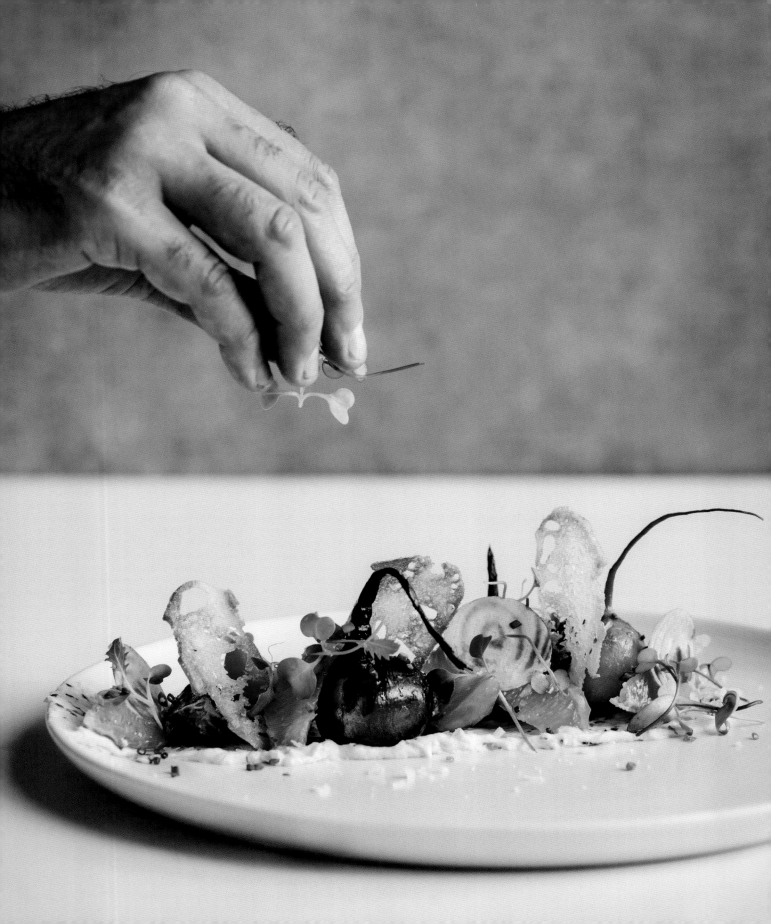

Pro Tip
You can make the olive dirt, eggs, and vinaigrette ahead and refrigerate for up to 2 days.

OLIVE DIRT

 MAKES A GENEROUS 1 CUP

½ cup halved pitted black olives

½ cup halved pitted Niçoise olives

¼ cup hazelnuts

1 tablespoon granulated onion

½ teaspoon mustard powder

1 Using a dehydrator set to high (about 155ºF), dry the black and Niçoise olives in a single layer on a rack until crisp, about 5 hours or overnight. You can also dehydrate the olives on a wire rack in a 160ºF to 170ºF oven with convection for about 5 hours.

2 Dry roast the hazelnuts on a baking sheet in a 375ºF oven until lightly browned, 8 to 10 minutes, shaking the pan once or twice. While still warm, rub off the skins in a paper towel.

3 Using a small food processor, spice grinder, or mortar and pestle, crush the dried olives to a fine meal the texture of dirt, shaking the processor as needed for even crushing. Transfer to a mixing bowl.

4 Add the roasted nuts to the processor, crush to a fine meal (the same texture as the olives), then transfer to the bowl. Mix in the granulated onion and mustard powder. Now you have tasty dirt. It will keep for a few months in a sealed container in the fridge.

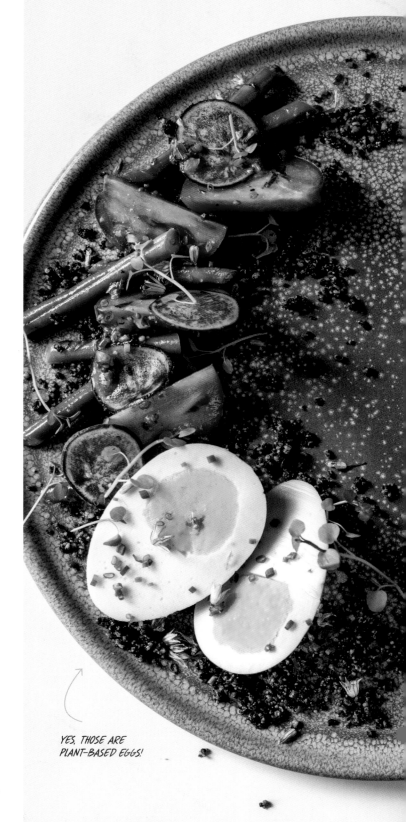

YES, THOSE ARE PLANT-BASED EGGS!

RECIPE CONTINUES →

PLANT-BASED EGGS

⬭ ⊕ **MAKES 8 TO 10 EGGS**

YELLOWS

½ cup dried potato flakes

¼ cup chickpea flour

3 tablespoons nutritional yeast

2 tablespoons red palm oil (see Pro Tips)

½ teaspoon fine kala namak (Indian black salt), plus more for garnish

½ cup hot water

WHITES

14 ounces silken tofu

1½ cups unsweetened soy milk

¾ cup water

1 teaspoon sea salt

1½ tablespoons mild-tasting oil, such as grapeseed oil

2 teaspoons agar powder

1 **FOR THE YELLOWS:** Whisk the potato flakes, chickpea flour, nutritional yeast, palm oil, and kala namak in a mixing bowl. Slowly whisk in the hot water. Stick the bowl in the fridge for a few minutes to firm up the mixture. Roll the mixture into oval balls about 1¼ inches in diameter with your hands. Chill the balls until ready to assemble the eggs.

2 **FOR THE WHITES:** Use a blender or food processor to blend the tofu, soy milk, water, and salt until smooth. Add the oil and blend slowly on the lowest setting. You want to avoid air bubbles in the whites. If it starts to bubble up, pour the mixture into a bowl, let it settle, then whisk in the oil by hand until blended.

3 Pour half of the white mixture into a small saucepan and heat over low heat. Add half the agar powder (1 teaspoon) and heat for 2 to 3 minutes, stirring gently to avoid creating air bubbles. The mixture should thicken to the consistency of thin pancake batter. Try to keep it from boiling, which could cause it to break and look grainy. If it breaks, remove the pan from the heat and whisk the mixture back together once it thickens up a bit.

4 Pour the mixture into large (the size of duck eggs) silicone egg molds (see Pro Tips), filling the bottom half of each. Chill until not quite firm, 10 minutes or so.

5 Meanwhile, repeat step 3 and cook the second batch of whites. Keep the white mixture warm in the pan.

6 For each mold, place a yellow ball a bit off center on top of a chilled bottom half of white, pressing gently. Put the lid on the mold, and use a funnel to slowly pour in more warm white mixture. Tap the mold to ensure the white mixture fills the inside of the mold. Chill until firm, about 30 minutes.

7 Gently remove the eggs from the molds by pushing the molds up from the bottom. Refrigerate the eggs in airtight containers for up to 2 days. Before serving, slice and sprinkle the eggs with about ½ teaspoon kala namak.

Pro Tips

→ We'll probably get shit for using palm oil here. See the second bullet point at Tal Ronnen's Pasta 101 on page 210 for more details on the controversy surrounding this healthy but potentially unsustainable fat. The bottom line is that there are better sources of palm oil than others. Nutiva brand gives 1% of their profits back to sustainable agriculture initiatives.

→ To shape the eggs, I use chocolate egg molds from Silikomart Professional. These are two-part egg molds with a hinge to make an entire egg that encloses the yellow center. Single half-egg molds will also work if you want to make egg halves. Just dig a hollow in the firmed-up whites and fit a halved yellow into each hollow.

KALE *and* AVOCADO SALAD *with* WILD RICE, GRAPES, *and* TOASTED SEEDS

For more than twenty-five years, the kale and avocado pairing has been one of my go-to combos. Some version of this dish has been served all over the world at every restaurant I have opened. It's now in almost every Whole Foods Market salad bar. It's just a slam dunk. The creamy fat in the avocado mellows out any bitterness in the greens, grapes add sweetness, lemons add acid, onions bring some sharpness, and rice and seeds give it nutty, earthy umami. Add ginger and cilantro if you like. Just keep in mind that kale, avocado, lemon, and salt are the foundation. From there, you can play around with whatever salad ingredients you like. —*CHAD*

 SERVES 2 TO 3

1 bunch kale (any type), stemmed and shredded fine (4 cups)

1½ cups cooked wild rice

½ cup small-diced red or yellow bell pepper

1 lemon, juiced

2 tablespoons flax oil or extra-virgin olive oil, optional

2 tablespoons thinly sliced green onions

½ teaspoon sea salt

1½ avocados, pitted, peeled, and diced

¼ cup halved small seedless grapes

¼ cup hemp, sesame, and/ or sunflower seeds, dry toasted

1 Grab a nice big mixing bowl, and toss in the kale, rice, bell pepper, lemon juice, oil (if using), green onions, salt, and avocado. If using oil, you can gently fold everything together. If you skip the oil, get some fat from the avocado by creaming it gently with your hands, massaging the avocado onto the greens. Fold in most of the grapes and toasted seeds, but save some for garnish.

2 Place on plates or in bowls and garnish with the reserved grapes and toasted seeds.

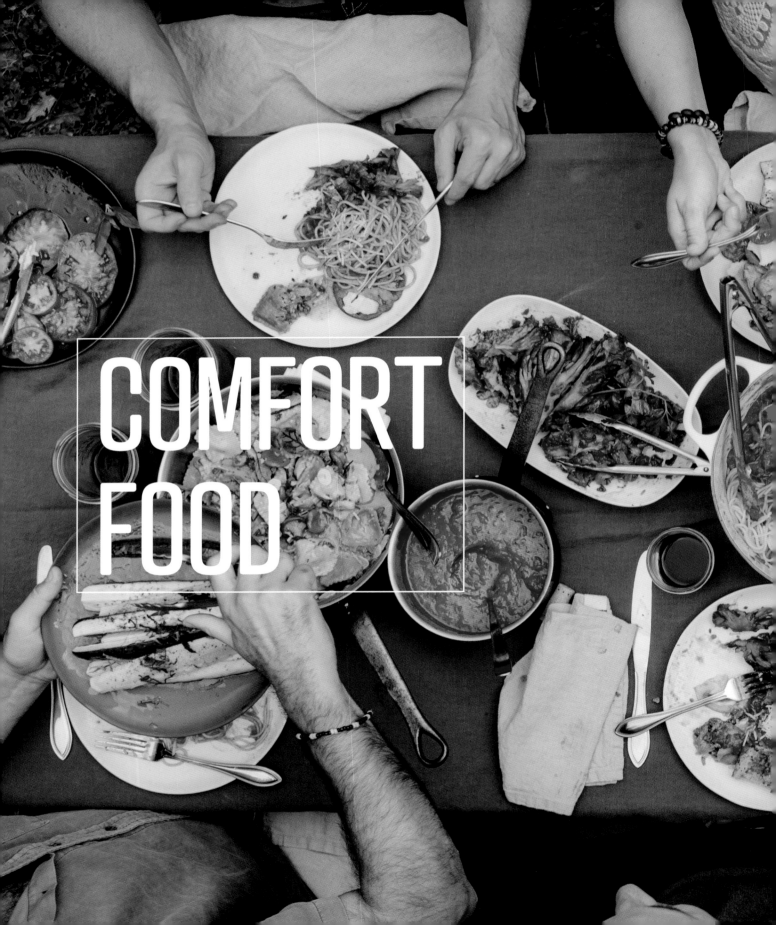

COMFORT FOOD

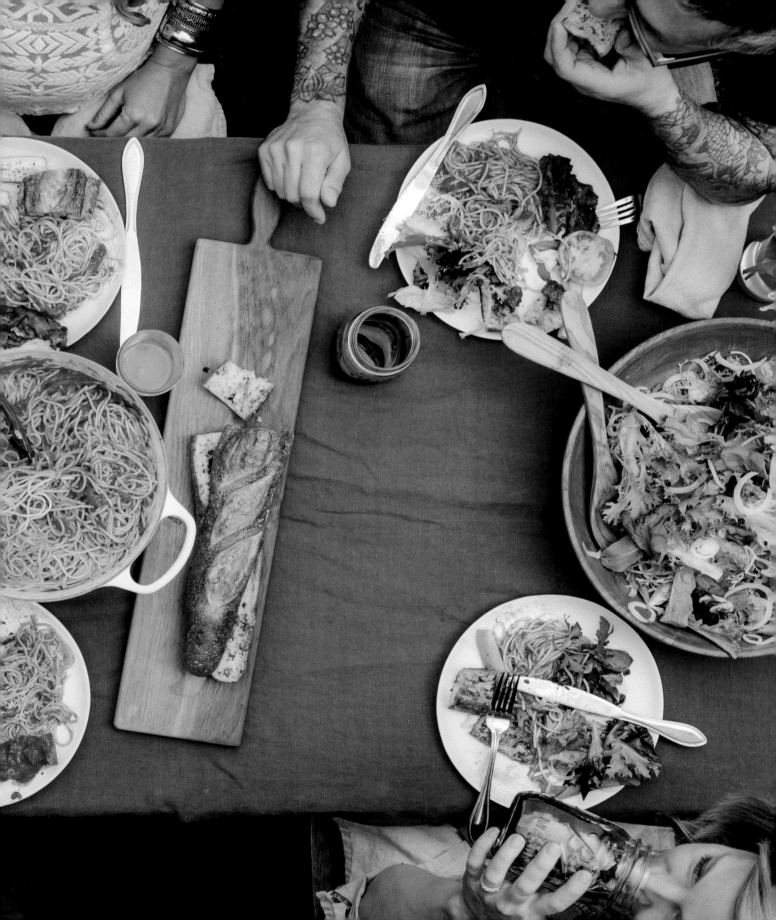

SPAGHETTI *with* NANA'S RED SAUCE

This is a Sarno staple that brings me back to my childhood. We pull it out whenever we need a quick meal. With garlic bread, salad, and a bottle of red, it's the perfect go-to dinner on weeknights. I could eat it five days a week. —*CHAD*

 SERVES 4

Nana Sarno's Red Sauce
   (page 265)
Sea salt
1 pound your favorite
   dried spaghetti or
   spaghettini

Chile flakes, optional
Chopped, fresh basil,
   optional
Plant-based Parmesan,
   such as from Follow
   Your Heart, optional

1   Be sure that Nana's sauce is in a pot on the stove on low heat.

2   Bring at least 1 gallon water to a boil in a large pot. Season the water with 2 tablespoons salt. (A large pot with plenty of water helps to keep the pasta from sticking, and the salt helps season the pasta and create a chewy yet tender al dente texture.) Add the pasta to the water, fanning it out. Give it a stir, then return the water to a boil and cook until the pasta is tender yet chewy when you bite into a piece, 8 to 10 minutes. Stir occasionally with tongs to prevent sticking. Strain in a colander. The sauce will cling to the pasta better if you don't rinse it.

3   There are two ways to serve spaghetti: Mix the pasta into the sauce in the pan, then transfer to a pasta bowl; or put the pasta in a bowl and pour the sauce on top. Most chefs like the former because you can meld the pasta and sauce together over low heat. But my kids pour their sauce on top because they don't like too much sauce. I'm not going to argue with them. Finish with a sprinkle of chile flakes, basil, and some Parmesan.

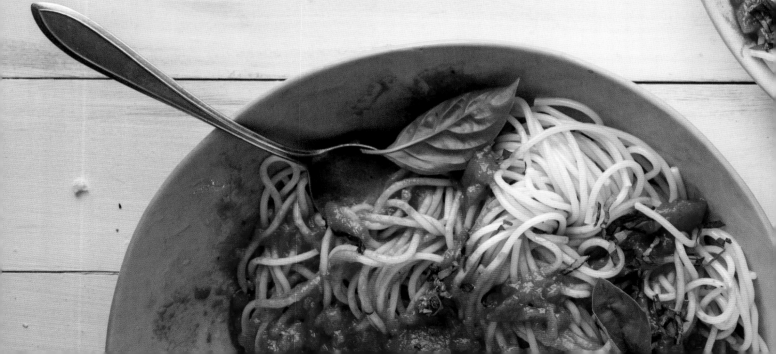

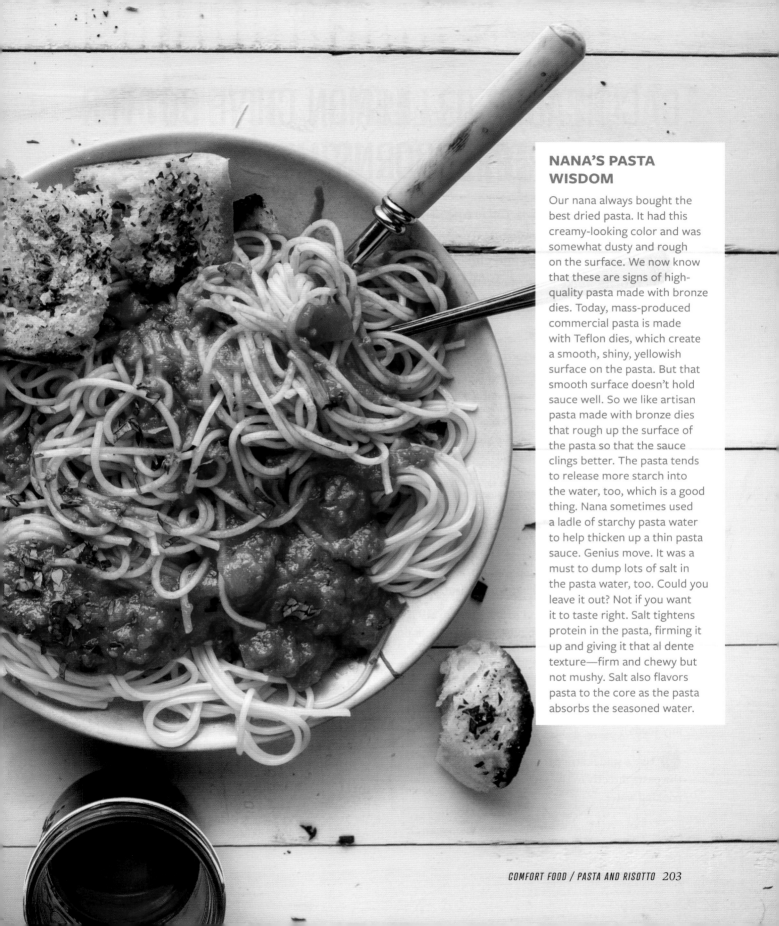

NANA'S PASTA WISDOM

Our nana always bought the best dried pasta. It had this creamy-looking color and was somewhat dusty and rough on the surface. We now know that these are signs of high-quality pasta made with bronze dies. Today, mass-produced commercial pasta is made with Teflon dies, which create a smooth, shiny, yellowish surface on the pasta. But that smooth surface doesn't hold sauce well. So we like artisan pasta made with bronze dies that rough up the surface of the pasta so that the sauce clings better. The pasta tends to release more starch into the water, too, which is a good thing. Nana sometimes used a ladle of starchy pasta water to help thicken up a thin pasta sauce. Genius move. It was a must to dump lots of salt in the pasta water, too. Could you leave it out? Not if you want it to taste right. Salt tightens protein in the pasta, firming it up and giving it that al dente texture—firm and chewy but not mushy. Salt also flavors pasta to the core as the pasta absorbs the seasoned water.

STROZZAPRETI *with* CAULIFLOWER MORNAY, MUSHROOMS, *and* KALE

Italians have some weird names for pasta. Linguine means "little tongues," orecchiette means "little ears," and strozzapreti means "priest-stranglers." No matter what you call this little twisted pasta, we say it's delicious—especially with a creamy white sauce dotted with mushrooms and kale. To get a jump on this bowl of comfort food, make the sauce a day or two ahead.

🍲 🍄 SERVES 6 TO 8

---

3 ounces dried wood ear mushrooms (black fungi)

1 bunch kale (about 1 pound), rinsed

1 pound strozzapreti or other short-shape dried pasta

2 tablespoons everyday olive oil

1 onion, diced

2 to 3 cloves garlic, thinly sliced

Cauliflower Mornay Sauce (page 262)

1 Soak the mushrooms in warm water to cover for 1 hour. Drain and rinse, then cut away any hard stems. Roughly chop the mushrooms and set aside.

2 Bring 1 gallon water to a boil in a large pot and season with 2 tablespoons salt.

3 Meanwhile, remove the ribs from the kale and tear the leaves into rough shreds. Set up a steamer and steam the kale until wilted, about 2 minutes. Remove from the heat and let cool a few minutes. Squeeze out any excess water, then roughly chop into bite-size pieces. Set aside.

4 Drop the pasta into the boiling water, give it a stir, and return the water to a boil. Cook until the pasta is al dente—tender yet chewy when you bite into a piece—8 to 10 minutes. Stir occasionally to prevent sticking.

5 While the pasta cooks, heat a large saucepot over medium-high heat. Add the oil, then the onion and garlic. Sauté for 2 minutes, then add the kale, 'shrooms, and Mornay. Heat until bubbling, about 2 minutes more.

6 Drain the pasta and add to the sauce. Stir and cook for another 2 minutes to meld pasta and sauce. Serve hot.

> **Pro Tip**
> *You can make the Mornay sauce a day or two ahead.*

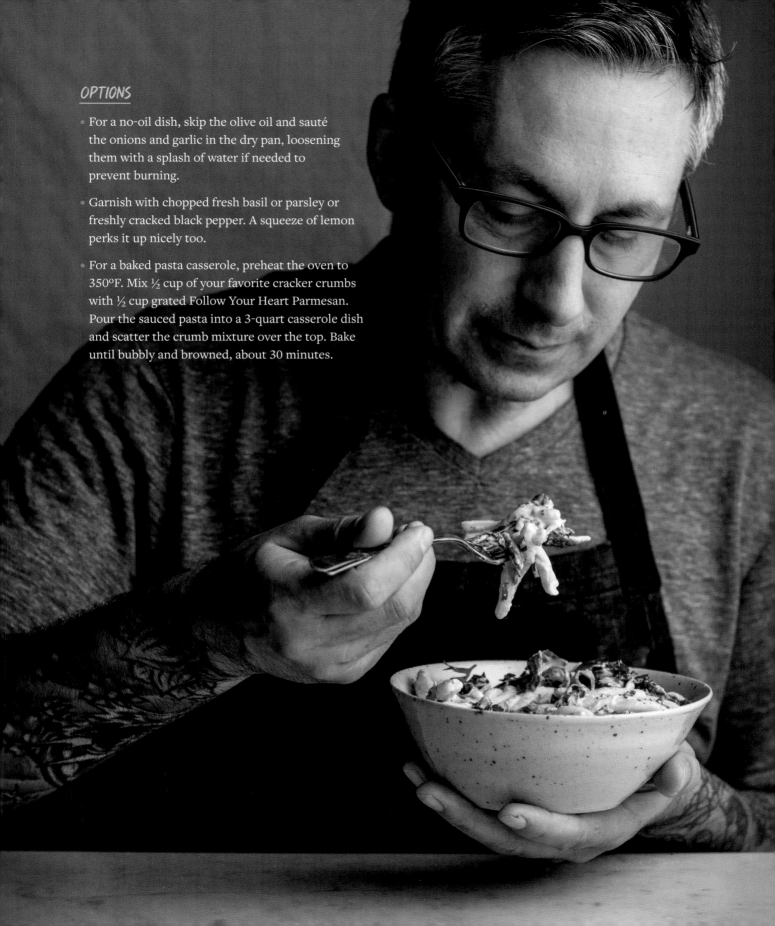

OPTIONS

- For a no-oil dish, skip the olive oil and sauté the onions and garlic in the dry pan, loosening them with a splash of water if needed to prevent burning.

- Garnish with chopped fresh basil or parsley or freshly cracked black pepper. A squeeze of lemon perks it up nicely too.

- For a baked pasta casserole, preheat the oven to 350°F. Mix ½ cup of your favorite cracker crumbs with ½ cup grated Follow Your Heart Parmesan. Pour the sauced pasta into a 3-quart casserole dish and scatter the crumb mixture over the top. Bake until bubbly and browned, about 30 minutes.

PASTA DOUGH

In March of 2013, I opened Crossroads Kitchen at the corner of Melrose and Sweetzer in Los Angeles. Crossroads is not what people picture when they think of a vegan restaurant. With upscale décor and lighting, we are the first plant-based restaurant in town to have a full bar. Most guests don't even make the connection that the menu is plant-based. We believe great food should be enjoyed by everyone at the table!

That belief is one of the things I have in common with Chad and Derek. I've known Chad for more than ten years. Over the years, I've gotten to know Derek as well. I've always admired Chad and Derek's cooking. We've had the pleasure of cooking together on several occasions, and I'm happy to share my fresh pasta recipe with them for this cookbook.

Although these directions are quite detailed, making fresh pasta dough is not at all difficult. A food processor mixes the dough quickly. Good pasta dough is firm, elastic, and easy to work with. Instead of eggs I use firm silken tofu, which adds protein and fat. It's virtually impossible to detect a difference between this and classic egg pasta dough. Note that silken tofu is sold in boxes and is shelf stable; you can usually find it in the produce aisle. You will need a pasta maker to roll and cut the pasta—either the manual kind or an attachment to your stand mixer. After resting, the dough can be rolled, cut, and cooked right away or refrigerated or frozen for future use. Allow the dough to come to room temperature before you roll it out. —*TAL RONNEN*

MAKES 1 POUND

½ (14-ounce) package firm silken tofu, drained

1½ cups "00" pasta flour, plus more as needed

1½ cups semolina flour, plus more as needed

3 tablespoons red palm oil

2 tablespoons filtered water, plus more as needed

½ teaspoon sea salt

1 Combine the tofu, flours, oil, water, and salt in the bowl of a food processor and process until the flour is evenly moistened and crumbly, about 10 seconds. Continue to process until the dough comes together to form a loose ball and feels moist but not sticky, about 2 minutes. Pinch the dough to test its consistency: If the dough seems excessively sticky, add more "00" flour, 1 tablespoon at a time, processing until just incorporated. If the dough is too dry, add a teaspoon or so of water. Dough is all about feel.

2 Remove the ball of dough from the food processor and wrap tightly in plastic wrap. (The food processor heats up the dough and makes it too soft to work with right away.) Refrigerate the dough for at least 1 hour to firm it up. The dough can be refrigerated for up to 1 day or frozen for up to 1 month.

3 Flour a work surface and your hands. Cut the dough into 4 equal pieces. Working with one piece at a time (cover the others to prevent them from drying out), roll or press the pasta out on a lightly floured work surface into a rough rectangle (image A). Feed the dough through the widest setting of a pasta machine; catch the sheet of dough in the palm of your hand as it emerges from rollers. Lightly dust both sides of pasta with a little flour. Run the dough through the machine two more times, then fold it into thirds.The dough will start to feel silky smooth. Then reduce the setting by one and crank the dough through again two or three times. Continue reducing the dial setting and rolling the dough through until the machine is at the second-to-narrowest setting (number 2 on most machines); the sheet should be about $\frac{1}{16}$ inch thick (image B). Cut the long sheet into two workable pieces, put them on a baking sheet dusted with flour and semolina, and cover with a damp towel. Repeat with the remaining pieces of dough.

4 The dough should be cut or shaped shortly after being rolled out so it won't dry out (image C). Or, to store the sheets of pasta, stack between pieces of wax paper, tightly wrap in plastic wrap, and freeze for up to 1 month.

OPTION

CHIVE PASTA DOUGH: Once the dough comes together in the processor, pulse into it 1 bunch of coarsely chopped chives (about ½ cup), just until you see green flecks throughout the dough.

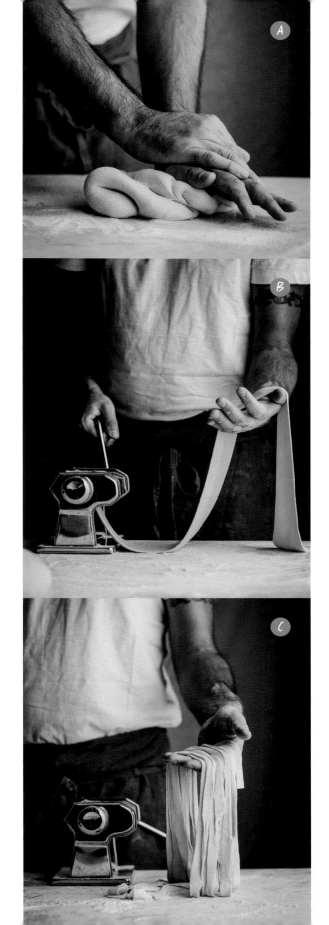

TAL RONNEN'S PASTA 101

▷ **Give yourself enough time and space.** Making fresh pasta is not difficult, but it does take time. Give yourself at least a couple of hours to make an entire batch—and rope a few friends or family members into helping if you can! Start with a clean countertop, and clear plenty of space to spread out as you work.

▷ **Use red palm oil.** Not to be confused with palm kernel oil, natural red palm oil is pressed from the fruit of the oil palm tree. Extremely high in antioxidants, it is regarded as one of the most nutritious oils in the world. It has a deep, rich orange-red color that gives this pasta dough an egg-yolk-yellow color. Palm oil originated in tropical West Africa, but it is now harvested in South America and Asia as well. Unfortunately, many of the palm trees grown commercially in other countries are extremely destructive to the environment and are threatening the rain forests. Be sure to purchase *only* unprocessed palm oil that comes from West Africa.

▷ **Use ample flour.** Pasta loves to stick to the baking sheet and to itself. Be sure to dust the baking sheet with a good amount of flour and semolina and lightly dust the dough too. And don't let filled pasta shapes touch each other once you've formed them.

▷ **Keep the dough covered.** Pasta dough dries out quickly if left uncovered, which makes it difficult to work with and prone to tearing. Work with one piece of dough at a time, keeping the dough you are not working with covered tightly with plastic wrap.

▷ **Don't overstuff the pasta.** It's tempting to overstuff pasta like tortellini and ravioli because what we like about them is the tasty filling. But overstuffing makes the pasta tricky to seal and can result in a dumpling that explodes in the boiling water. Practice restraint, and stick to the amount of filling specified in the recipe.

▷ **Bring a pot of heavily salted water to a rolling boil.** A generous amount of salt in the water seasons the pasta internally as it absorbs liquid and swells. As a result, your pasta dish may require less salt overall.

▷ **Do not add oil to the cooking water.** Oil added to the cooking water will coat the pasta and keep the sauce from adhering to it. The sauce won't be absorbed and, as a result, the pasta will be flavorless.

▷ **Return the water to a boil quickly.** After you add the pasta, keep the heat on high to bring the water back to a boil as quickly as possible (put a lid on the pot if necessary). Then cook the pasta, uncovered, at a fast boil.

▷ **Stir during the first minute or two of cooking** to prevent sticking. This is the crucial time, when the surface of the pasta is still coated with sticky, glue-like starch. If you don't stir, the pieces of pasta can stick together. Frequent stirring with a wooden spoon will ensure the pieces move freely and help the pasta cook evenly.

▷ **Do not rinse.** Rinsing the pasta after draining cools the pasta and prevents it from absorbing the sauce; the starch remaining on cooked pasta helps the sauce cling. Just drain the pasta in a large colander standing in the sink, then shake it well to remove excess water.

▷ **Use the cooking water.** It's always a good idea to reserve a bit of the cooking water when you drain the pasta to stir into the sauce. The small amount of starch left in the cooking water can thicken your sauce slightly while loosening it at the same time.

▷ **Do not oversauce.** Toss pasta with just enough sauce to coat it to avoid a big puddle on the bottom of the plate. It's always best to add the pasta to the sauce, not the other way around.

PORCINI RAVIOLI *with* GARLIC BUTTER *and* SORREL

I'm often asked what I serve to people new to eating plant foods. Fresh pasta! Stuff it with some meaty porcini mushrooms and no one leaves the table hungry. I like fall porcinis better than spring ones. They're more aromatic—almost floral. Spring porcinis tend to taste a little musty and minerally, but either works. Adding some plant-based butter deepens the rich, earthy taste, and sorrel brightens everything up. There are a few components here, so save this dish for a special dinner. You won't be disappointed. —*CHAD*

 SERVES 4 TO 5

PORCINI RAVIOLI

2 tablespoons plant-based butter

1½ tablespoons everyday olive oil

3 tablespoons minced white onion

3 cloves garlic, minced

1 pound fresh porcini mushrooms (see Pro Tips), minced

1½ teaspoons minced fresh thyme

½ cup white wine

2½ tablespoons porcini powder (ground dried porcini; see Pro Tips, page 212)

Sea salt and freshly ground black pepper

2 tablespoons Kite Hill cream cheese

Pasta Dough (page 208), prepared through step 3

SAUCE AND PLATING

1 tablespoon everyday olive oil

4 ounces wild mushrooms, halved or whole

Sea salt

3 tablespoons plant-based butter

3 tablespoons diced shallots or white onions

3 cloves garlic, minced

½ cup white wine

1½ cups Mushroom Stock (page 284)

2 tablespoons chopped fresh chives

Freshly ground black pepper

Fresh baby sorrel, for garnish

1 *FOR THE FILLING:* Heat a medium sauté pan over medium-high heat. Add the butter and oil, heat until the butter melts, then add the onion and garlic. Sauté until the onion is golden, 3 to 4 minutes. Add the fresh mushrooms and thyme. Cook, stirring occasionally, until the mushrooms begin to stick to the pan, 6 to 8 minutes. Pour in the wine, scraping the pan bottom, then lower the heat to medium and stir in the porcini powder. Cover and cook until the mushrooms break down and most of the liquid evaporates, 8 to 10 minutes.

2 Taste the filling and add salt and pepper until it tastes good to you. Transfer to a mixing bowl and stir in the cheese until incorporated. Let the filling cool while you roll out the pasta.

3 Lay a pasta sheet on a lightly floured surface and use a 1-ounce (2-tablespoon) scoop to drop mounds of filling about 1 inch apart in two rows down the center of the dough.

RECIPE CONTINUES →

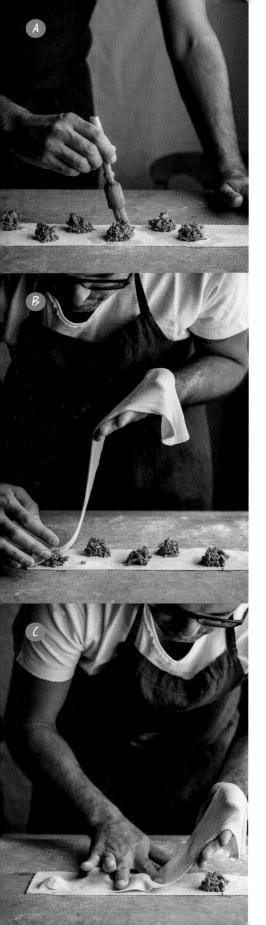

4 Dip your finger in water or use a pastry brush to moisten each long side of the dough (image A). Carefully lay another pasta sheet over the dough and filling (image B). Press the dough around the filling to remove any air pockets (image C). Dust a round, square, or other shape ravioli cutter that's about 3 inches wide. Press out each ravioli and place on a floured baking sheet. Place the pan in the refrigerator or freezer.

5 Repeat rolling, filling, and pressing out the ravioli with the remaining dough and filling. Refrigerate the ravioli until ready to use, or up to 6 hours.

6 *FOR THE SAUCE*: Heat a medium sauté pan over medium-high heat. Add the oil and when hot, place the mushrooms in the pan in a single layer and sear until golden, 2 to 3 minutes per side. Remove to a plate.

7 Bring a large pot of water to a boil and season with salt (a generous teaspoon per quart of water).

8 Add the butter to the same hot sauté pan and when it melts, add the shallots and sauté until golden brown, 3 to 4 minutes. Add the garlic and cook 1 minute. Return the seared mushrooms to the pan, then add the wine and simmer until the wine mostly evaporates, about 2 minutes. Add the stock and cook until the liquid reduces in volume by about half, 2 to 3 minutes.

9 Cook the ravioli in the boiling water until they float to the top, about 3 minutes. Remove one and taste it to make sure the pasta is tender, but avoid overcooking. This pasta can actually get chewier if you overcook it.

10 Use a slotted spoon or spider strainer to lift the pasta from the water and transfer it to the pan of sauce. Add the chives, then season with some salt and pepper. Shake the pan to meld everything together.

11 Remove from the heat and divide among warm plates. Garnish with a scattering of sorrel.

Pro Tips

→ *If you can't find porcini mushrooms, use the same amount of cremini (baby bella) mushrooms, but increase the amount of porcini powder to ⅓ cup to boost the porcini flavor.*

→ *To make porcini powder, just grind dried porcini mushrooms in a spice grinder or clean coffee mill.*

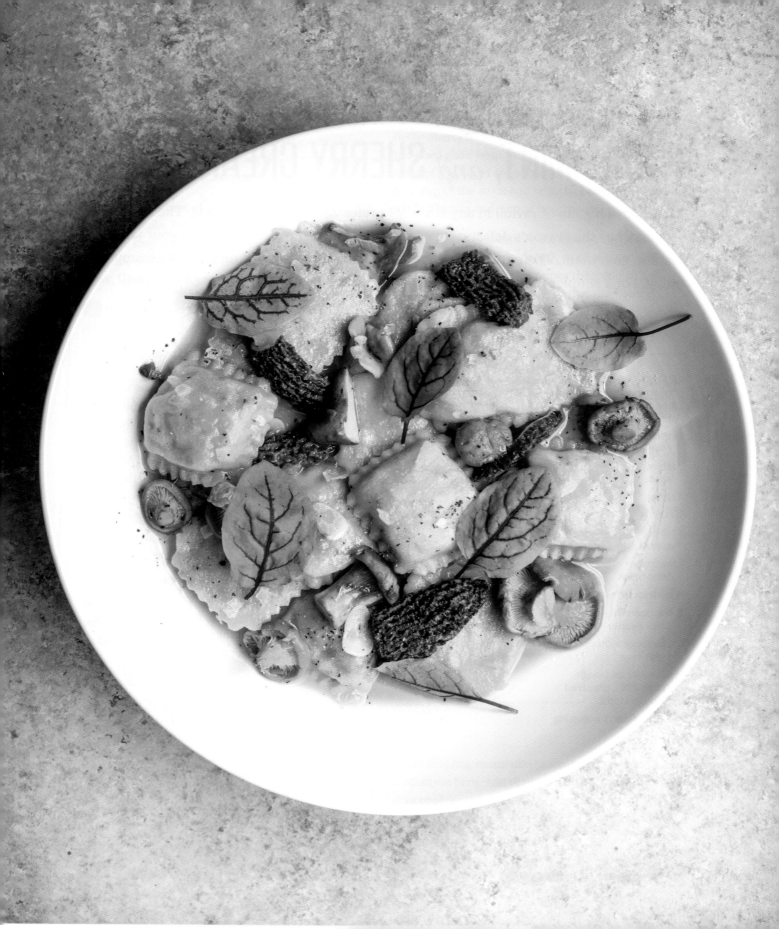

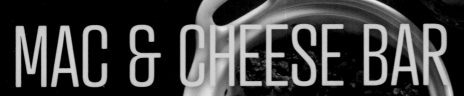

MAC & CHEESE BAR

PUT OUT SOME TOPPINGS AND BOWLS, AND INVITE A HALF DOZEN OF YOUR FRIENDS OVER. IT'S A MAC PARTY!

BASES
Mac & Cheese (see Options on page 261)
Baked Mac & Cheese (page 261)

THIS ONE'S MADE WITH GEMELLI

CREAMY
Additional Wicked Healthy Cheese Sauce (page 260)
Cauliflower Mornay Sauce (page 262)

YES, PLEASE!

SAVORY
Sliced and pan-seared mushrooms of any kind
Crumbled and pan-seared Field Roast sausage

SEASON WITH SALT AND PEPPA

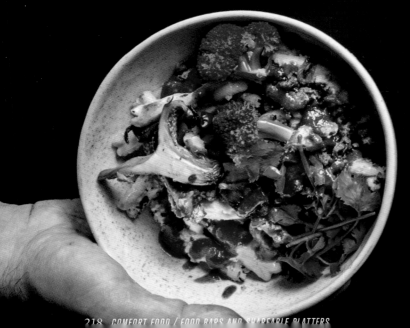

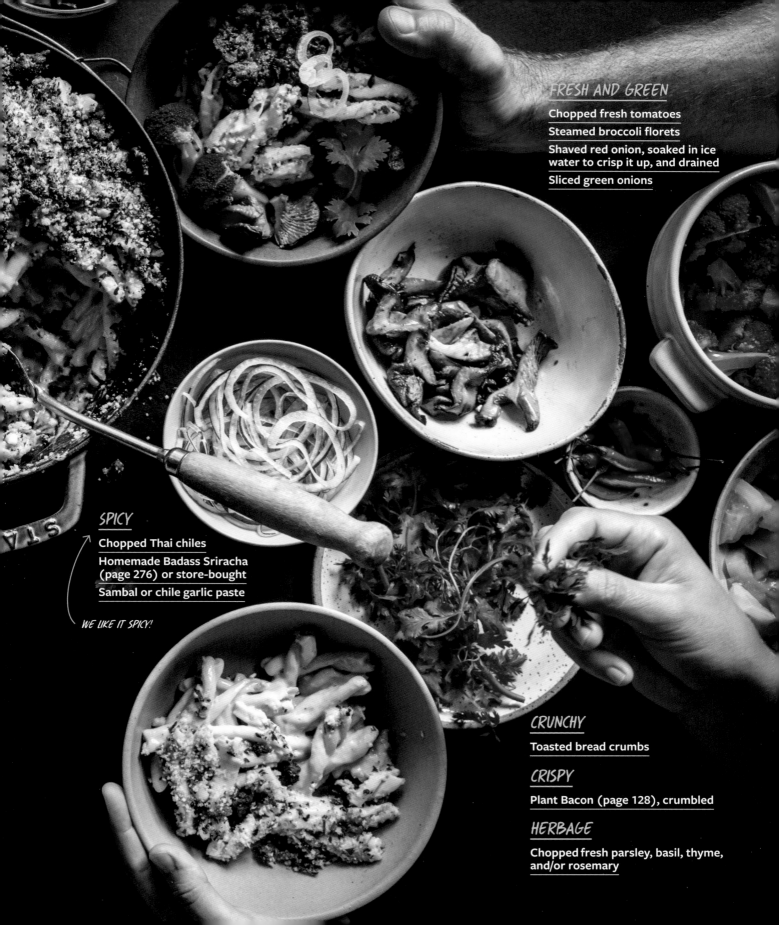

FRESH AND GREEN

Chopped fresh tomatoes

Steamed broccoli florets

Shaved red onion, soaked in ice water to crisp it up, and drained

Sliced green onions

SPICY

Chopped Thai chiles

Homemade Badass Sriracha (page 276) or store-bought

Sambal or chile garlic paste

WE LIKE IT SPICY!

CRUNCHY

Toasted bread crumbs

CRISPY

Plant Bacon (page 128), crumbled

HERBAGE

Chopped fresh parsley, basil, thyme, and/or rosemary

LOADED BAKED POTATO BAR

A classic baked potato is one of the easiest, most satisfying dishes out there. For a potato bar, make a bunch and set them out with the toppings and options below.

Russet potatoes, scrubbed, pricked with a fork, and baked naked at 375°F for 1 hour

Field Roast Italian or Mexican chipotle sausage, broken up and pan-seared in a little oil

TO MAKE THE SAUSAGE BITS EXTRA-CRISPY, SEAR IN AN OVEN-SAFE PAN, THEN BAKE WITH THE POTATO FOR 20 MINUTES.

Steamed or roasted broccoli florets

Wicked Healthy Cheese Sauce (page 260)

Sliced green onion

BETTER YET, USE ALL 3.

OPTIONS

- Brush the spuds with oil before baking for a crisp skin.

- Use sweet potatoes instead of russets.

- Instead of sausage, use a few tablespoons crumbled Plant Bacon (page 128) or roasted mushrooms.

- Instead of broccoli, go for steamed or roasted cauliflower florets.

- Add diced grilled asparagus.

- Add some herbage like chopped fresh cilantro, parsley, thyme, and/or rosemary.

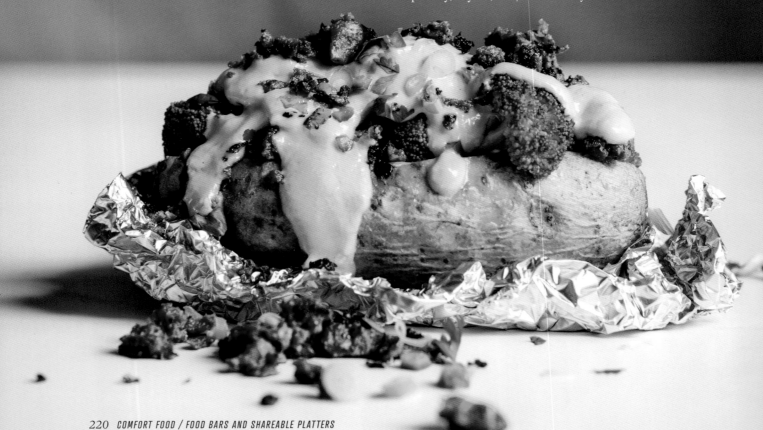

STUFFED AVOCADO BAR

Avocados are rich, creamy, and healthy. What's not to love? Bake them with our cheese sauce, set them out with optional toppings, and let about a half dozen guests pile on their favorite flavors. Here are some possibilities.

Small avocados, halved and pitted

Wicked Healthy Cheese Sauce (page 260)

Hot Chocolate Lentils (page 108)

Heirloom Tomato Salsa (page 274)

Poached Corn Salsa (page 275)

Carrot Habanero Citrus Hot Sauce (page 278)

Fresh herbs like parsley and cilantro, or some microgreens

1 Preheat the oven to 350ºF.

2 Carve out a little extra space in each avocado half with a spoon, then fill the hole with cheese sauce. Place the filled avocados on a baking sheet and bake until heated through, 10 to 15 minutes.

3 Put out your toppings and let your guests dig in!

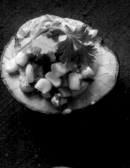 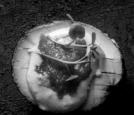 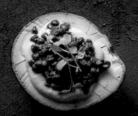 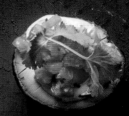

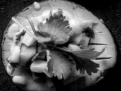 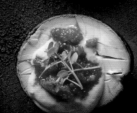 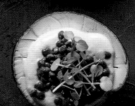 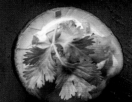

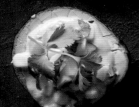 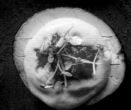 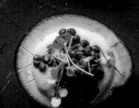 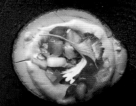

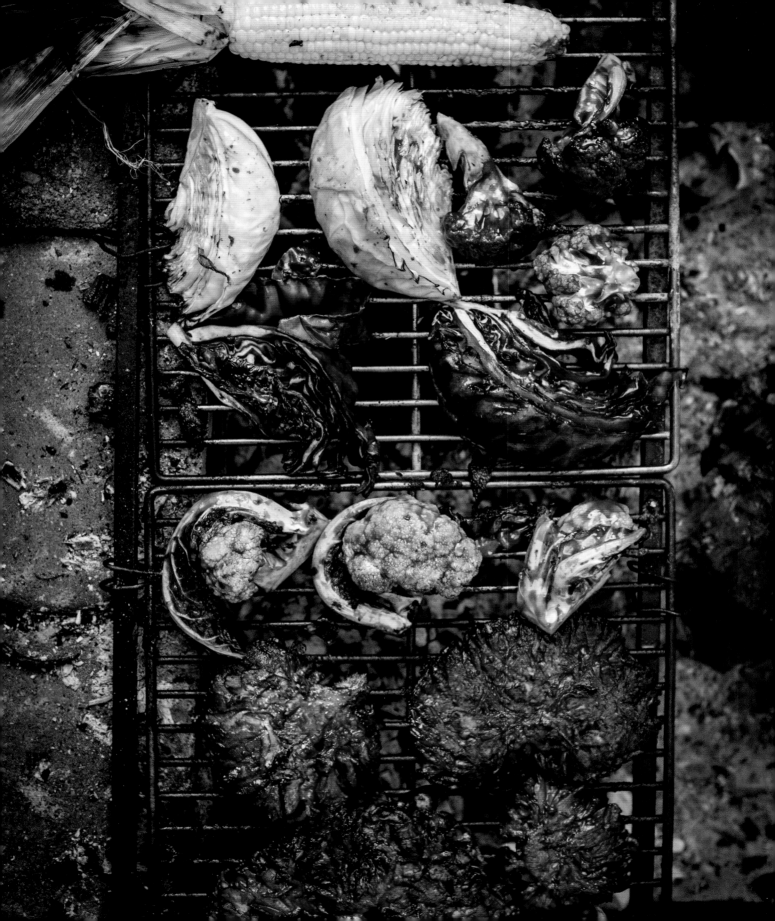

BARBECUED MAITAKE STEAKS

This is a deeply satisfying plant-pusher dish—truly eye-opening for hard-core meat eaters. When you press and sear a big, fluffy maitake mushroom, it develops a dense, meaty texture and satisfying browned flavor. Then you can barbecue it low and slow with some wood chunks or chips, and baste it with barbecue sauce. Take your pick from the three BBQ seasoning and sauce options on page 224: smoky Texas, spicy Korean Bulgogi, or Asian-inspired char siu. You can also use the steaks to make four or five Spicy Maitake Steak Sandwiches (page 123). —*DEREK*

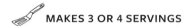 **MAKES 3 OR 4 SERVINGS**

---

4 tablespoons peanut oil or vegetable oil (or red palm oil for char siu barbecue)

1 pound maitake mushrooms (6 to 10 whole mushroom clusters; see Pro Tips, page 224), cleaned

Texas, bulgogi, or char siu barbecue seasoning (page 224)

Texas, bulgogi, or char sui barbecue sauce (page 224)

1 Heat a large heavy pan (such as cast iron) over medium heat until very hot, about 2 minutes. Add 1 tablespoon of the oil, swirling to coat the pan. Add half of the mushroom clusters and use a second heavy pan or a couple of foil-wrapped bricks to weight down and press/sear the mushroom clusters. Cook for 2 minutes, then remove the weight and the mushrooms to a work surface.

2 Add another 1 tablespoon oil to the pan, swirling to coat. Flip the mushrooms and season the cooked side with half of the seasoning. Return the mushrooms to the hot pan, raw-side down. Return the weight to the mushrooms and press/sear the other side. Cook for 2 minutes, then remove the weight and flip the mushrooms in the pan. Season the newly cooked side with the remaining seasoning.

3 Return the weight to the mushrooms and cook another 2 minutes. Repeat this process of flipping, weighting down, and searing the clusters until the mushrooms are condensed and pressed into crispy golden brown steaks with almost no liquid left in the pan, about 10 minutes total. Poke the mushrooms to test whether they are finished cooking. They should feel compact yet fleshy, the way the fleshy base of your thumb feels when you poke it while firmly making the okay sign. Repeat with the remaining oil and mushrooms.

4 When the 'shroom steaks are compact and golden brown, remove them to a baking sheet. Brush generously with a thick layer of sauce on both sides and let marinate at room temperature for at least 1 hour. Or, if you have time, marinate in the refrigerator for up to 2 days. The longer you marinate, the more flavor you'll get.

5 To barbecue the steaks, heat a charcoal grill or smoker to medium low, 250ºF to 350ºF (or see Pro Tips, page 224, to roast in the oven). Push the coals or wood to one side to keep the heat to one side of the grill only. Throw a wood chunk or a few handfuls

RECIPE CONTINUES →

of wood chips onto the edge of your charcoal fire. Put the steaks on the opposite, cooler side of the grill, then put down the lid. Cook slowly until the mushrooms are heated through and charred here and there, 30 to 40 minutes total. Every 10 minutes, flip the steaks and brush with sauce so all sides are glazed with a thick layer. If the steaks threaten to burn, lower the heat by closing the air vents or move the steaks to a cooler part of the grill.

6 Remove the barbecued steaks to a cutting board and let rest for 5 minutes. Slice on an angle to create wide slices. You can also leave the steaks whole and refrigerate them for up to 4 days before using.

> **Pro Tips**
> → *Maitake mushrooms (a.k.a. hen-of-the-woods) grow in big clusters. Buy the biggest clusters you can find and keep them whole. Or use oyster mushrooms. Oysters are more watery, so be patient: They'll take longer to firm up when you press and sear them. You could even use giant portobello mushroom caps—minus the stems.*
>
> → *If you don't have a grill or smoker, you can roast the seared mushroom steaks on a baking sheet at 400°F, turning and basting with the sauce until the mushrooms brown here and there, 30 to 40 minutes total.*

TEXAS BARBECUE

TEXAS SEASONING

½ tablespoon sea salt

½ teaspoon freshly ground black pepper

¼ teaspoon smoked paprika

¼ teaspoon ground cumin

¼ teaspoon chili powder

¼ teaspoon granulated garlic

¼ teaspoon granulated onion

¼ teaspoon mustard powder

TEXAS SAUCE

2 cups prepared BBQ sauce, like Austin's Own

½ cup beer, like Deschutes Mirror Pond Ale (drink the rest)

¼ cup Marshall's Haute Sauce Carrot Curry Habanero, or another carrot curry hot sauce

BULGOGI BARBECUE

BULGOGI SEASONING

½ tablespoon sea salt

1 teaspoon freshly ground black pepper

1 teaspoon granulated onion

BULGOGI SAUCE

1 cup Ninja Tamari Glaze (page 267) or straight-up tamari

1 cup hoisin sauce

¼ cup toasted sesame oil

3 tablespoons brown rice syrup

1 tablespoon minced garlic

1 tablespoon minced ginger

1 tablespoon black sesame seeds, for sprinkling on at the end

1 tablespoon white sesame seeds, for sprinkling on at the end

CHAR SIU BARBECUE

CHAR SIU SEASONING

½ tablespoon sea salt

1 teaspoon freshly ground black pepper

1 teaspoon granulated onion

CHAR SIU SAUCE

1 cup tomato paste

½ cup Ninja Tamari Glaze (page 267) or straight up tamari

OR 3 TABLESPOONS RICE VINEGAR COMBINED WITH 1 TABLESPOON BROWN RICE SYRUP (OR AGAVE) AND ½ TEASPOON CELERY SALT

½ cup beet juice, preferably fresh pressed (see Pro Tip, page 190)

¼ cup Homemade Badass Sriracha (page 276) or other sriracha

¼ cup hoisin sauce

¼ cup Pok Pok Som Chinese celery drinking vinegar

1 tablespoon minced garlic

½ teaspoon smoked paprika

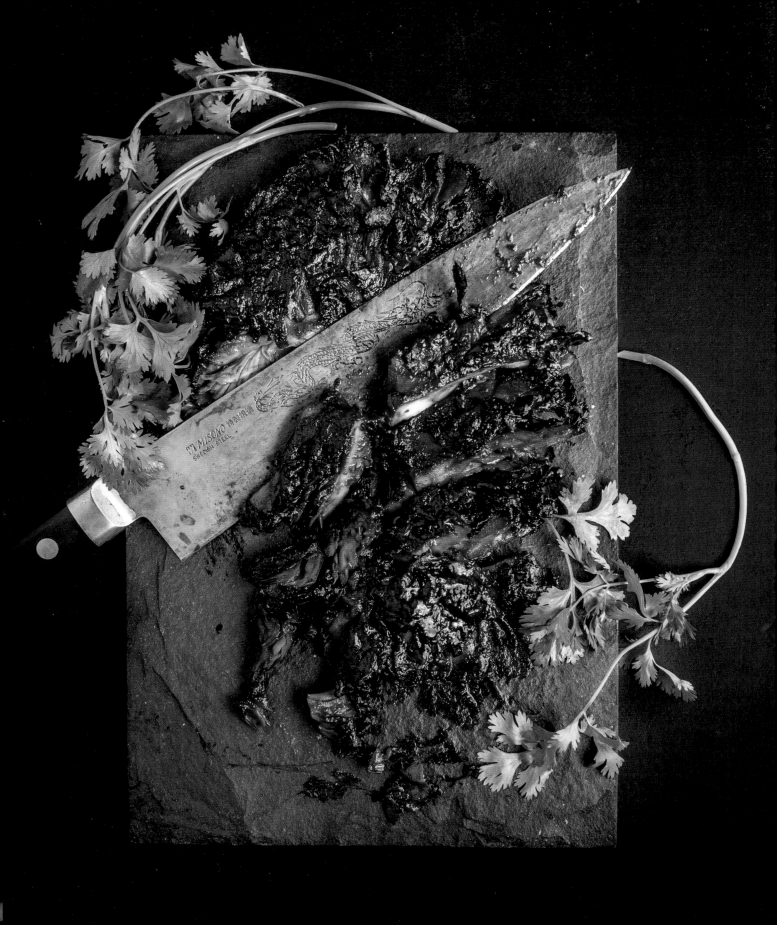

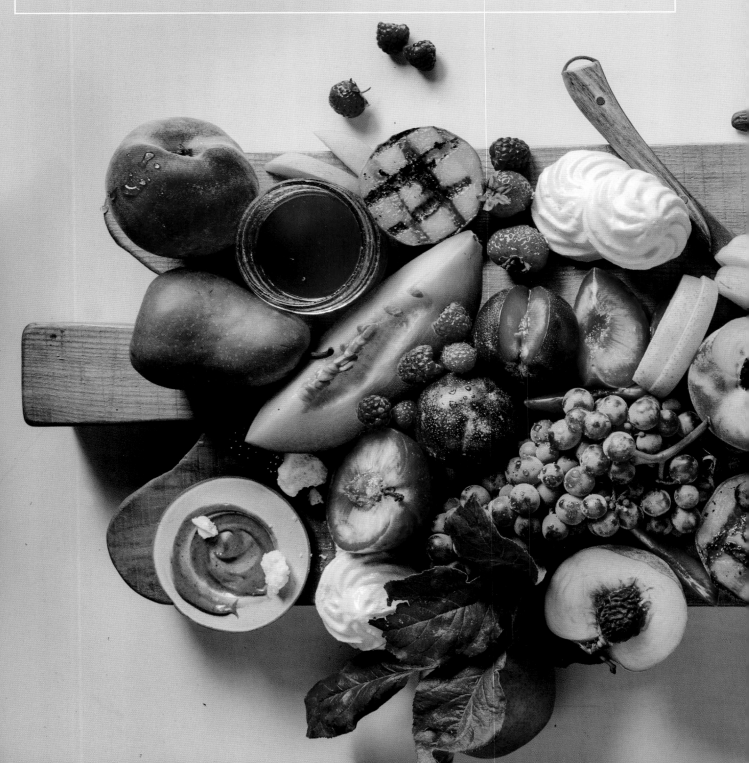

NATURE'S CANDY

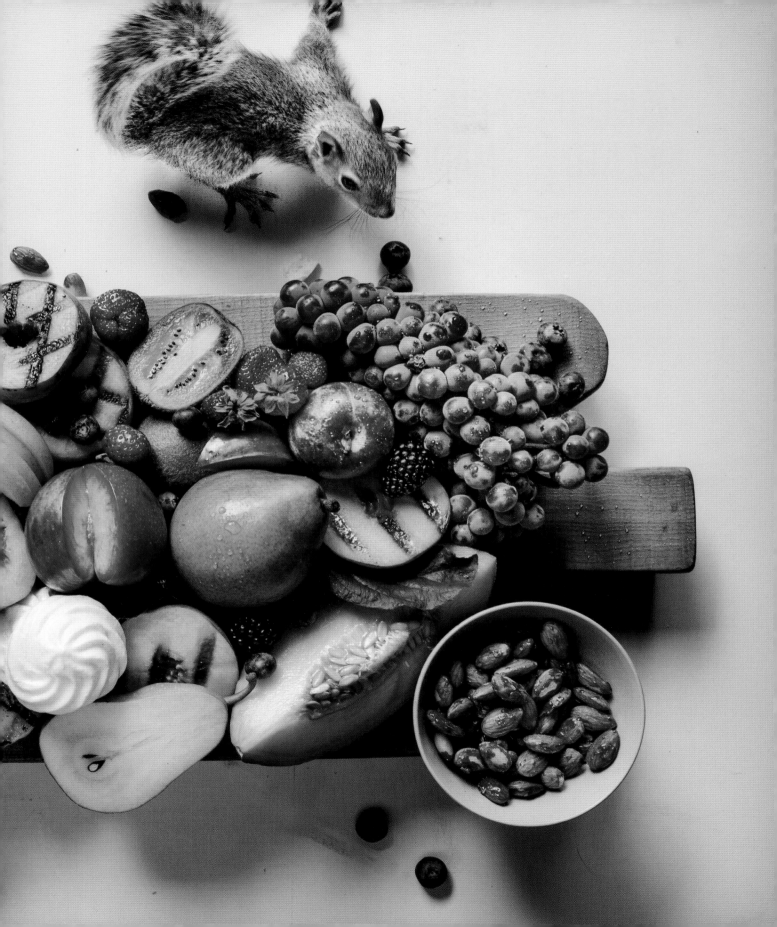

GRILLED PEACHES *with* VANILLA SPICED GELATO *and* MANGO SRIRACHA CARAMEL

We served this dessert to Martha Stewart in May of 2013 and she absolutely loved it. Walter Robb, the co-CEO of Whole Foods Market, had a dinner party in Austin, and Martha was the guest of honor. Mango Sriracha Caramel, the real star of the dish, adds a spicy, sweet, savory, and bright finish. The ultimate flavor bomb. The caramel, paired with grilled ripe peaches and spiced gelato, hits all the taste buds from every direction. It's Martha-worthy!

 SERVES 8 (HALF A PEACH EACH)

3 tablespoons good-quality white balsamic vinegar

3 tablespoons agave syrup or other liquid sweetener

2 tablespoons hot water

1 tablespoon walnut oil or olive oil

Pinch of freshly ground star anise

4 ripe but not too soft peaches, halved and seeded

2 cups Vanilla Spiced Gelato (page 229)

½ cup Mango Sriracha Caramel (page 270)

1 Heat a grill (or grill pan) to high heat.

2 Whisk together the vinegar, agave, water, oil, and star anise. Using a pastry brush, brush the mixture on the flesh side of the peaches.

3 When the grill is hot, reduce the heat to medium. Scrape the grill grate clean. Place the peaches flesh-side down on the grate and grill until nicely browned, about 3 minutes. Brush some glaze over the top as they cook. If you're using a grill pan inside, make sure your fan is on or a window is open. There will be some smoke here.

Remove the peaches from the grill and set on plates. Serve each with ¼ cup gelato and a drizzle of the sriracha caramel.

OPTION

• Want some added crunch? Finish this dish with Ninja Nuts (page 52) or your favorite salted and roasted or candied nuts.

VANILLA SPICED GELATO

 MAKES ABOUT 1 QUART

1 cup raw cashews

1 can (14 ounces) full-fat coconut milk

¾ cup nondairy milk

¼ cup agave syrup or other liquid sweetener

Seeds scraped from 1 split vanilla bean

½ teaspoon vanilla extract

½ teaspoon freshly grated ginger

½ teaspoon freshly ground black pepper

¼ teaspoon ground star anise

¼ teaspoon nutmeg

Pinch of sea salt

½ teaspoon guar gum

LOOK FOR GUAR GUM IN THE NATURAL FOODS SECTION OF THE GROCERY STORE.

1 Soak the cashews overnight in water to cover. Drain and place in a high-speed blender. Add everything else except the guar gum and blend on high speed until smooth, 1 to 2 minutes. When smooth, continue blending and add the guar gum with the machine running (this prevents clumping). Blend for a few seconds.

2 Freeze the mixture in an ice cream maker, following the manufacturer's directions. (They're all a little different. We love the simplicity of the KitchenAid frozen ice cream bowl attachment.) Pack into containers, cover, and freeze for up to 1 month.

OPTION

• For a wicked whipped cream, whip the gelato instead of freezing it. Add ⅓ cup additional nondairy milk to loosen it, then whip on medium-high speed until fluffy, 3 to 4 minutes; or whisk vigorously by hand, 5 to 6 minutes. The texture should be soft like shaving cream.

5 Line a couple of baking sheets with parchment paper, using a small dollop of meringue under each corner to hold down the parchment.

6 Use an offset spatula to spread the berry meringue in an even layer over the parchment in each pan. Make the layer no thicker than ¼ inch.

7 Bake the meringue until firm to the touch, about 1¼ hours, rotating the pans once or twice for even cooking.

8 Let the berry paper cool completely in the pans. When cooled, break the meringue into shards and seal in an airtight container. It's crucial to store these meringues in an airtight container. Room temperature is fine, but any humidity will turn them from crisp to sticky almost immediately. Stored in a cool, dry place, they'll keep for weeks. In a hot and humid place, they'll turn sticky in a day or two—even if kept in a container.

9 *FOR THE PINEAPPLE MERINGUE*: Buzz the freeze-dried pineapple in a small food processor or clean coffee mill to a fine powder, then measure out ⅓ cup. Return the reserved meringue to the mixer, and whip in the ⅓ cup pineapple powder and the vanilla until fully incorporated. Scrape into a pastry bag or zipper-lock bag and snip off a corner.

10 *MAKE THE PINEAPPLE BRÛLÉE*: Peel, core, and slice the pineapple into 12 rectangles, each about 2 inches long and 1 inch wide.

11 Melt the butter in a large sauté pan over medium heat. Stir in the sugar until it dissolves, then stir in the rum and a splash of water. Cut the heat to low and add the pineapple in a single layer. Simmer gently just until the pineapple is glazed and lightly browned all over but not turned to mush, turning a few times to brown all sides. Remove the pan from the heat and set aside.

12 *TO ASSEMBLE*: Gather 4 to 6 large white plates. On each one, spoon a couple of tablespoons of spiced panko off center in a straight line. Arrange 3 to 4 pieces of pineapple near the panko. To brûlée the pineapple, use a kitchen torch to broil the tops. This step is optional but it adds good char flavor.

13 Grab the bag of pineapple meringue and squeeze 4 to 5 small dollops of meringue in between the pineapple pieces. Place a few fresh berries in between the pineapple on the panko. Arrange a few shards of berry paper over the top and serve.

Pro Tips

→ *You can buy whole or powdered freeze-dried fruit from karensnaturals.com.*

→ *Look for pure vanilla powder in gourmet stores or online. You want pure powder that's not mixed with powdered sugar.*

→ *You'll have some meringue left over. It can be made into cookies—just follow the baking directions for Almond Meringue Cookies (page 236).*

OPTION

• For a gluten-free dessert, replace the panko with gluten-free panko, ground toasted almonds, or other nuts.

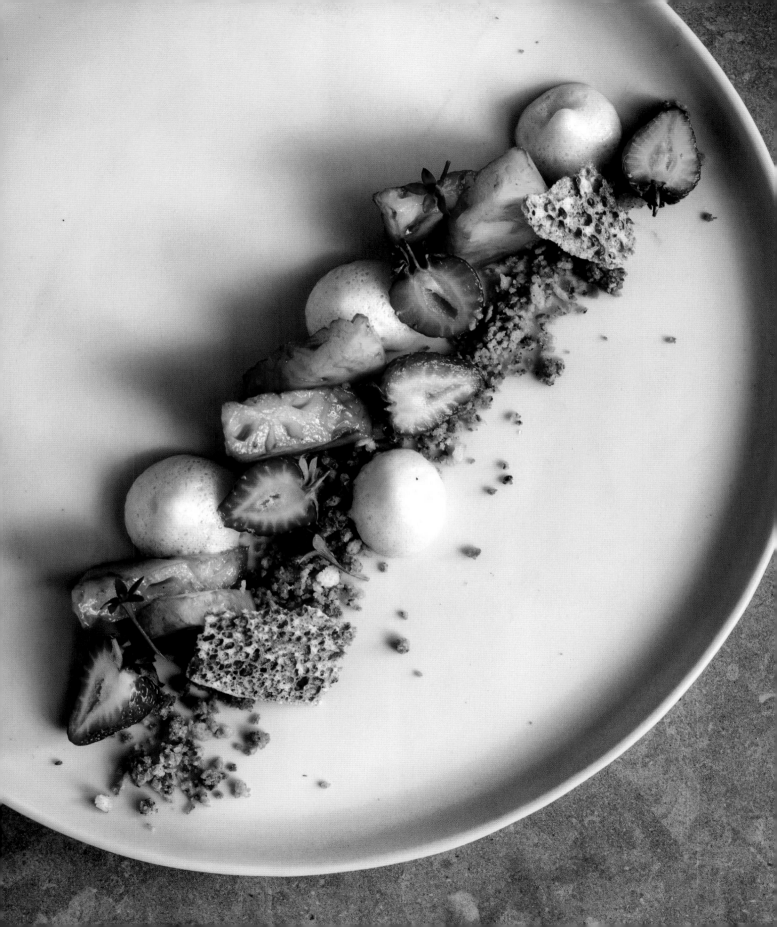

PLANT-BASED MERINGUE

This recipe still blows our minds. You mean the leftover liquid from a can of beans (called aquafaba) can be used to make desserts?! Most people pour their bean liquid down the drain. But surprise—it has enough protein to whip up just like egg whites. *Voilà*—plant-based meringue! You can use this meringue as a base for everything from pancakes and pastries to meringue-topped pies and Almond Meringue Cookies (page 236). All without a hint of beany-ness. You can even use aquafaba to make Plant-Based Mayo (page 264).

 MAKES 6 TO 7 CUPS MERINGUE

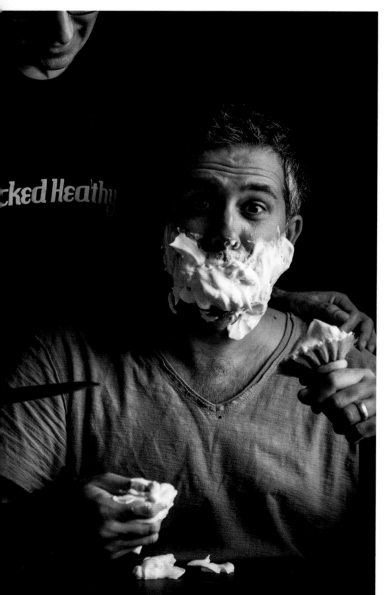

1 can (14 ounces) no-salt-added chickpeas

½ teaspoon cream of tartar

½ cup semifine (see Pro Tip) organic cane sugar

1 Strain the chickpea liquid into the bowl of an electric mixer. You should have about ½ cup. (Use the chickpeas for something else such as the Four-Bean and Sweet Potato Slow-Cooker Chili on page 166).

2 Add the cream of tartar to the bowl and fit the mixer with the whisk attachment. Whip on high speed until the mixture increases in volume and stiffens a bit, 4 to 6 minutes.

3 Reduce the speed to medium high and gradually add the sugar, a few tablespoons at a time. Blend about 4 minutes more, stopping and scraping down the sides of the bowl as necessary. The meringue is done when it holds its shape as the whip attachment is lifted. You should also be able to hold the bowl upside down without the meringue falling out. Continue whipping until you can do that. Otherwise, the meringue will not hold its shape when cooked.

> **Pro Tip**
> *To make semifine sugar, grind it in a food processor or Vitamix for 10 to 15 seconds.*

MERINGUE 101

▷ We recommend using a stand mixer here. This needs to whip for a looooong time—10 to 12 minutes—a little too much time for you to hold a handheld mixer.

▷ You might be tempted to cut down the amount of sugar, but we don't advise it. This amount helps to cut the bean flavor.

▷ The bean liquid should start out with a consistency like loose egg whites...sorta gelatinous looking. If your bean liquid is watery, boil it in a pan until it's thicker and reaches that egg white-y consistency. Cool before using.

▷ In general, 2½ tablespoons of bean liquid = 1 egg white.

▷ This meringue is temperamental, so use caution if adding alcohol or acids like citrus juice or vinegar. In order for the meringue to set properly when baked, the cream of tartar will need to be adjusted so that the total acid in the mixture is properly balanced.

▷ Use the meringue as soon as possible. Within a day of refrigeration, it will begin to deflate, break down, and leak liquid.

▷ For more information and for common FAQs about this cool ingredient, be sure to check out aquafaba.com.

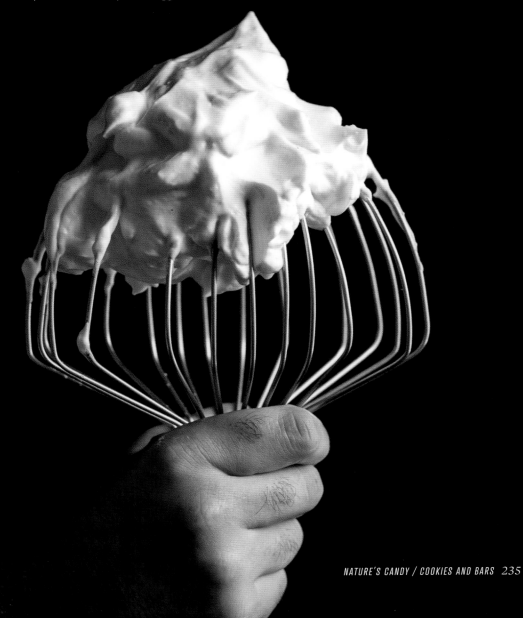

ALMOND MERINGUE COOKIES

In the fall of 2015, we featured these cookies on several catering menus. We usually made them with dried fruit powder like raspberry, then dried the meringue in sheets and broke it up into shards, as in Brûléed Pineapple with Spiced Panko, Berries, and Meringue (page 231). Flavor the cookies however you like (see the Options), but try to stick with freeze-dried fruit powders. Liquid extracts and flavorings tend to make the meringues fall. —CHAD

 MAKES ABOUT 50 SMALL COOKIES

Plant-Based Meringue
(page 234)

1 teaspoon almond
extract

Seeds scraped from
½ vanilla bean

¼ cup finely ground
unsalted roasted
almonds, optional

1 Preheat the oven to 200°F. Line two baking sheets with parchment paper.

2 Make the meringue until it is fully whipped. Whip the almond extract and vanilla seeds into the meringue.

3 Spoon the meringue into a pastry bag fitted with a round tip. Or use a zipper-lock bag and cut off a corner. If your parchment is curling up from the baking sheets, dollop a little meringue under each corner to secure it. Pipe cookies into pointy mounds about 1½ inches in diameter. They should look like big Hershey's kisses. You need only about ½ inch space between cookies because they won't expand much during baking. Sprinkle the ground almonds, if using, evenly over the cookies.

4 Bake until the cookies look dry and off-white in color, 2 hours. Rotate the pans halfway through the baking for even heating. Cool completely on the baking sheets. Store in well-sealed containers. Humidity and moisture will make the cookies sticky, so store them in a cool, dry cupboard.

OPTIONS

RASPBERRY MERINGUE COOKIES: When making the meringue, add ⅓ cup powdered freeze-dried raspberries (buzzed in a clean spice grinder) along with the sugar. Omit the vanilla and almonds, and substitute raspberry extract for the almond extract.

LEMON MERINGUE COOKIES: When making the meringue, add 2 tablespoons lemon peel powder (buzz the dried lemon peel in a clean spice grinder) along with the sugar. Omit the vanilla and almonds, and substitute lemon extract for the almond extract.

CANDY CANE MERINGUE COOKIES: When making the meringue, reduce the sugar by 2 tablespoons and add 3 to 4 tablespoons crushed candy canes along with the sugar while whipping. Omit the vanilla and almonds, and substitute 1 teaspoon peppermint extract or a few drops of food-grade peppermint essential oil for the almond extract.

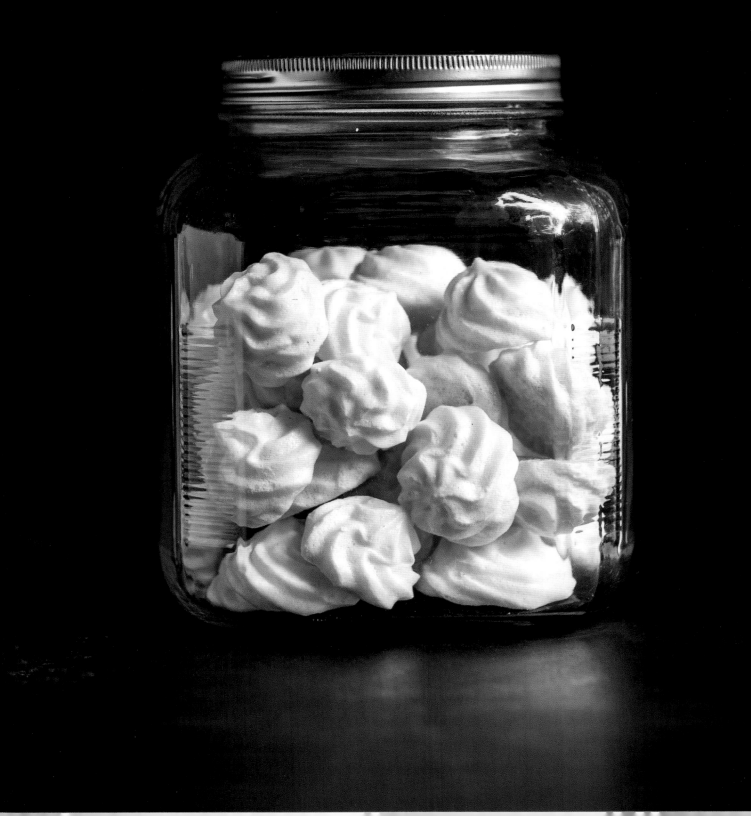

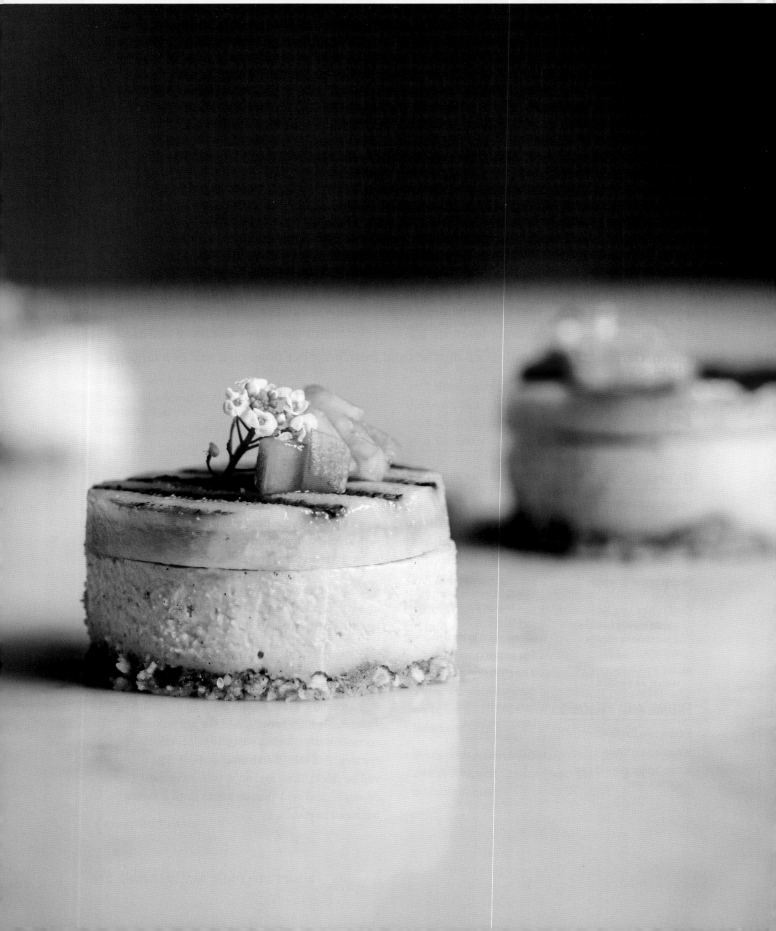

5 Spoon the filling over the crust and freeze until set, at least 1 hour. You can also cover and keep the cheesecake frozen for up to a month.

6 *FOR THE PEACHES:* Pit the peaches by cutting lengthwise around and down to the pits. Twist apart the halves and discard the pits. Slice the peaches into ¼-inch-thick rounds. Spray the slices on both sides with spray oil to help prevent sticking.

7 Heat a grill pan over high heat (or light an outdoor grill). When hot, grill each slice until marked with deep brown stripes, 2 to 3 minutes per side. Remove to a cutting board and cool slightly. Use a ring mold or round cookie cutter that is slightly smaller than the peach slices (2- to 3-inch diameter) to cut the peaches into perfect rounds.

8 If frozen solid, thaw the cheesecake until it's just cold. Cut the whole cake into slices or punch out rounds as shown in the photo. (See Pro Tips for ways to use the scraps of cheesecake.)

9 *TO ASSEMBLE:* Place a round of cheesecake on each plate and top with a grilled peach round. Drizzle the lavender syrup on the plate around the cheesecake just before serving.

Pro Tips

→ *If you can't find lucuma powder, you could use 1 cup crushed graham crackers.*

→ *Enjoy the leftover scraps of cheesecake as snacks, or layer them up into a trifle with fresh berries and Plant-Based Whipped Cream (page 244).*

KABOCHA TART *with* SALTED ALMOND CRUMBLE *and* ESPRESSO SYRUP

A bold twist on classic pumpkin pie, this dessert explodes with flavor—especially in the salted almond crust and espresso syrup drizzle. For the filling, I pureed roasted kabocha squash and baked the puree naked like a flan. That way, you can serve only as much crust as you want, treating it more like a nutty crumble to complement the filling. Let's call it deconstructed pumpkin pie. If you can't find kabocha squash, use buttercup or butternut. Make this dessert more wicked with some Plant-Based Whipped Cream (page 244) and a scoop of Amaretto Gelato (page 230).

 SERVES 6 TO 8

SQUASH FILLING

2½ pounds kabocha squash

Coconut oil, for the pan

1 cup full-fat coconut milk

⅓ cup maple syrup

½ cup coconut sugar

6 tablespoons cornstarch

1 tablespoon pumpkin pie spice

1 teaspoon finely grated or minced fresh ginger

1 teaspoon vanilla extract

½ teaspoon ground cinnamon

½ teaspoon sea salt

ALMOND CRUMBLE

1 cup almonds

¼ cup raw turbinado sugar

1 tablespoon flake salt, such as Maldon

Pinch chipotle chile powder, optional

Espresso Syrup (page 243)

1 **FOR THE FILLING:** Preheat the oven to 400°F. Halve the squash and remove the seeds and strings. Cut the squash into small pieces and place the pieces face-down on a rimmed baking sheet. Put the pan in the oven and pour enough hot water into the pan to barely cover the bottom. Roast until the squash is fork-tender, 50 to 60 minutes, and remove from the oven.

2 Drop the oven temp to 350°F, and lightly oil a 9-inch square baking pan with coconut oil.

3 Scoop the softened flesh from the squash skins into a food processor or high-speed blender and puree. You should have about 2¼ cups squash puree. Add the remaining ingredients to the puree and blend until super smooth.

4 Pour the mixture into the prepared baking pan and spread evenly. Bake until the filling begins to pull away from the sides of the pan (the middle of the filling may crack slightly), about 1 hour. Let cool to room temperature (about 1 hour). Then chill until cold, at least 2 hours. It will keep in the fridge for up to a week.

5 **FOR THE CRUMBLE:** Toast the almonds in a sauté pan over medium heat, shaking the pan now and then, until the nuts are lightly browned and smelling nutty, about 2 minutes. Turn out into a bowl and let cool.

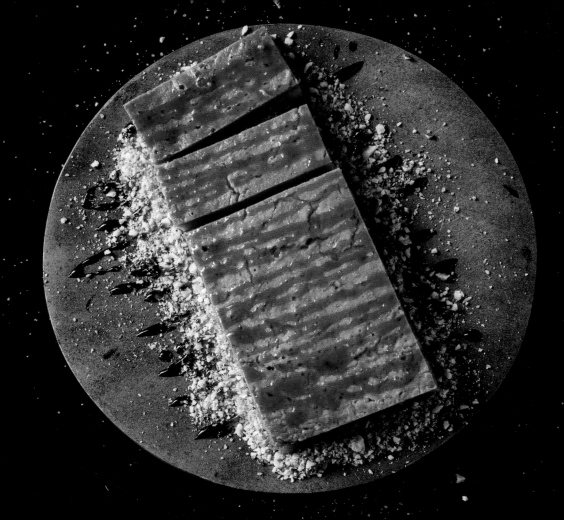

6 Transfer the cooled almonds to a food processor and add the sugar, salt, and chipotle (if using). Process until reduced to crumbs, but be careful not to take it all the way to nut butter. Transfer to a bowl. This sweet and salty crumble keeps for weeks. It's great sprinkled on almost any dessert.

7 *TO ASSEMBLE:* Place a generous amount of the almond crumble on each of 6 to 8 dessert plates. Slice the chilled pie filling into 12 to 16 slices. Carefully remove each slice of filling and place two on top of each crumble serving. Drizzle with espresso syrup. You can assemble the crumble and filling on one large platter, as shown in the photo.

ESPRESSO SYRUP

 MAKES ABOUT 1 CUP

1 cup good-quality brewed espresso

1 cup maple syrup

½ cup water

1 vanilla bean, split

Pinch of sea salt

Put everything in a small saucepan and bring to a boil over high heat. Cut the heat to low and simmer until the liquid gets syrupy and reduces in volume by about half, 20 to 25 minutes total. The finished syrup should coat the back of a spoon while still hot. Remove from the heat and let cool completely. Use immediately or refrigerate for up to 1 week. Just don't eat the vanilla bean.

PLANT-BASED WHIPPED CREAM

This recipe comes from David Joachim, our badass collaborator. Dollop it on everything from cake and brownies to fresh fruit to your partner's nipples. Yum.

 MAKES ABOUT 1¼ CUPS

1 can (14 ounces) full-fat coconut milk

1 to 2 tablespoons organic cane sugar

1 teaspoon vanilla extract

1 Chill the unopened coconut milk can in the fridge for 8 hours or overnight. Chill a whip attachment or whisk and metal mixing bowl in the freezer for 10 minutes before you whip the cream.

2 Open the can—without shaking it—and carefully spoon out the white coconut cream from the top into the chilled mixing bowl, leaving the clear coconut juice in the can. Use the leftover coconut juice to flavor cocktails.

3 Add the sugar and vanilla to the mixing bowl and whip on medium-high speed until fluffy, 3 to 4 minutes; or whisk vigorously by hand, 5 to 6 minutes. The texture should be soft like shaving cream. Avoid overwhipping or the cream will eventually go from creamy to grainy.

4 Use immediately or cover and refrigerate for a few hours. Re-whip as necessary to keep it fluffy.

Pro Tip

To stabilize the cream so it stays fluffy for more than a few hours, evenly scatter ⅛ teaspoon xanthan gum over the mixture at the beginning of whipping.

OPTIONS

- Swap the cane sugar for agave syrup, maple syrup, or honey.

- Use other flavor extracts like almond, orange, or peppermint.

- You can replace the 14-ounce can of coconut milk with half of a 14-ounce can of pure coconut cream, available in some grocery stores.

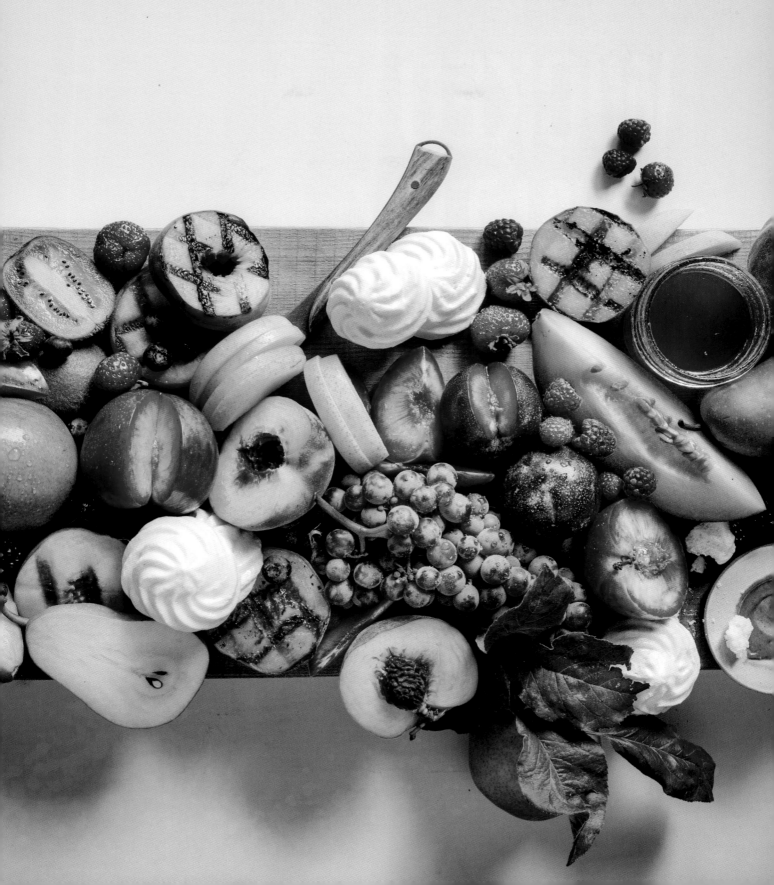

WICKED HEALTHY JUICES AND COCKTAILS

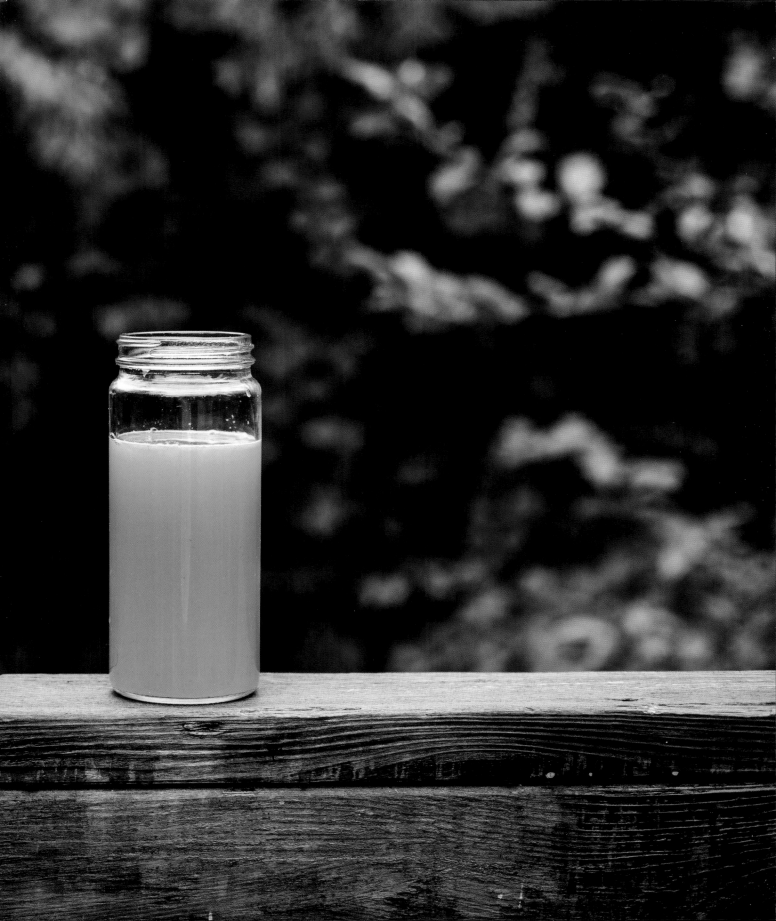

WICKED HEALTHY JUICES

Anytime your body needs a shot of healthy goodness, make some fresh juice. To make any of the juices here, first rinse all your ingredients and then cut them to fit your juicer. Juice it all up and toss it back while the juice is fresh. If you don't have a juicer, as a last resort, you could use a blender instead. But keep in mind that the blender's friction and heat may destroy some of the nutrients, and the resulting juice will be pulpier—more like a thin smoothie than juice. In that case, strain out the pulp for a thinner juice.

CUCUMBER, CELERY, GREEN APPLE, and KALE JUICE

 MAKES 2 BIG GLASSES

1 large cucumber

3 stalks celery

Handful stemmed kale

Handful stemmed spinach

½ to 1 Granny Smith apple, cored and quartered (skip the apple if you like your juice less sweet)

½ lemon, peeled (or squeezed if using a blender)

SPICY PINEAPPLE, SPINACH, KALE, and LIME JUICE

 MAKES 2 BIG GLASSES

1 pineapple, peeled, cored and cut into spears for juicing (about 3 cups)

1 green jalapeño chile, halved and seeded

Handful stemmed spinach

Handful stemmed kale

1 lime, peeled (or squeezed if using a blender)

IRON MAN JUICE

 MAKES 2 BIG GLASSES

1 red beet

1 cup spinach

2 seedless oranges, peeled (or squeezed if using a blender)

1 red bell pepper, halved and seeded

1 big slice peeled fresh ginger (½ inch thick)

WICKED HEALTHY COOLERS

When you're hot and sweaty, cool off with a refreshing drink made from real fruit. To make any of these coolers, first muddle your fruit, herbs, aromatics, and citrus in a carafe or bar shaker. Crush 'em up good to release maximum aroma. Then stir in any other juices, the sweetener, and filtered water, if using (hold off on any soda water for now). Cover and shake it all up—or stir like a whirling dervish. Taste a spoonful and add more sweetener or juice until it tastes good to you. Pour over ice in a tall glass and add soda water, if using that instead of filtered water. For a party, make a giant batch and serve in a clear glass dispenser. Feeling wicked? Add 1 to 2 ounces vodka per glass.

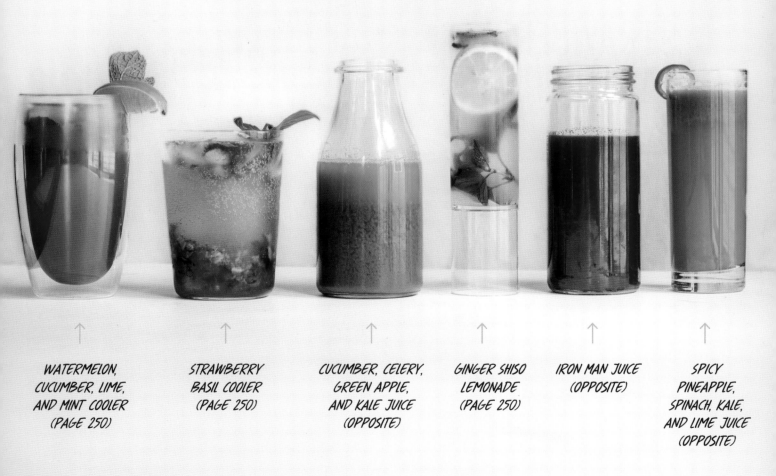

↑
WATERMELON, CUCUMBER, LIME, AND MINT COOLER (PAGE 250)

↑
STRAWBERRY BASIL COOLER (PAGE 250)

↑
CUCUMBER, CELERY, GREEN APPLE, AND KALE JUICE (OPPOSITE)

↑
GINGER SHISO LEMONADE (PAGE 250)

↑
IRON MAN JUICE (OPPOSITE)

↑
SPICY PINEAPPLE, SPINACH, KALE, AND LIME JUICE (OPPOSITE)

GINGER SHISO LEMONADE

 SERVES 4

3 large fresh shiso leaves (or 8 fresh basil leaves)

3 slices fresh ginger (about ¼-inch-thick coins)

4 lemons, juiced, Meyer lemons preferred

3 tablespoons agave syrup or other sweetener

4 to 5 cups cold filtered water

STRAWBERRY BASIL COOLER

 SERVES 4

½ cup fresh strawberries, stemmed and rinsed

4 large basil leaves

2 lemons, juiced, Meyer lemons preferred

3 tablespoons agave syrup or other sweetener

4 to 5 cups soda water

WATERMELON, CUCUMBER, LIME, *and* MINT COOLER

 SERVES 4

1 large cucumber, juiced in a juicer

Small handful mint leaves

1 tablespoon agave syrup (optional, if watermelon is not sweet enough)

1 lime, juiced

4 cups watermelon, juiced in a juicer

1 to 2 cups soda water

Thin slices lime and/or cucumber, for garnish

INFUSION COCKTAILS

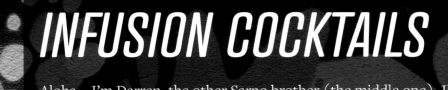

Aloha—I'm Darren, the other Sarno brother (the middle one). I've been tending bar for twenty-five years. I started in college, mostly at the Sea Ketch in Hampton Beach, New Hampshire, where we grew up. After college, I moved to Maui and tended bar all over the island. When Derek and Chad told me they were writing a book, I wanted in. I dreamed of infusing spirits with the fruits and spices they use in their cooking. We could infuse whiskey, tequila, vodka, and gin with whole spices like vanilla beans, star anise, and Thai chiles. We could make flavored syrups with fresh aromatics like ginger and lemongrass. I also came up with an all-purpose fresh lemon sour mix—so much better than packaged dry sour mix.

To make any of the infused spirits called for here: Combine the spirits and spices in a 16-ounce Mason jar, seal, and let them sit at room temperature for 12 to 36 hours (the full 36 for the strongest infusion). Strain out the spices and your cocktails are just a few shakes away. Each infusion makes 12 ounces, which is enough for several cocktails and keeps indefinitely at room temperature. Oh, and each cocktail recipe makes 1 drink. If you're serving more, just double or triple (or quadruple) the amounts. —DARREN

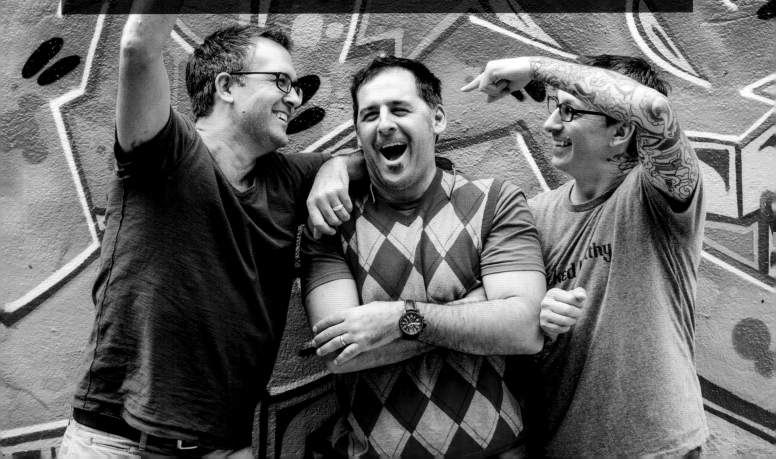

CITRUS *and* SPICE

With tequila, chiles, and fresh grapefruit juice, this spicy drink smacks of South Texas. But ginger syrup takes it closer to Asia. For a sexy rim, mix together a 1:1 combo of fine sea salt and demerara or brown sugar on a plate. Run a lime wedge around the rim of the glass, then dip the rim in the salt-sugar mix to coat. —*DARREN*

 SERVES 1

2 ounces Chile Citrus Tequila

½ ounce Ginger Syrup

2 ounces freshly squeezed grapefruit juice

Ice

Soda water

Pour the infused tequila, ginger syrup, and grapefruit juice in a shaker tin. Add the ice and shake vigorously for 10 seconds. Strain over crushed ice in a tall collins glass. Top with the soda water.

> **Pro Tip**
> *If you're new to the cocktail game, grab a vegetable peeler. It's the best tool for making a citrus swath, which is a wide strip of citrus zest cut from the peel. The thin blade of the peeler lets you strip off a wide swath of the aromatic citrus zest without the bitter white pith underneath.*

Chile Citrus Tequila

12 ounces 100% blue agave blanco tequila

2 whole Thai chiles

3 swaths lemon zest

3 swaths lime zest

Seal in a Mason jar for 12 to 24 hours.

Ginger Syrup

1 cup water

1 cup organic cane sugar

7 slices fresh ginger (about 1-inch diameter each)

Simmer in a saucepot until the syrup thickens (8 to 10 minutes), then strain and cool. Refrigerate for up to 1 month.

SARNO SAZERAC

A classic Sazerac gets anise aromas from absinthe. To switch things up, I infuse the rye whiskey with star anise instead. Orange bitters add a sexy twist. For a lighter, less wicked drink, pour it over an ice sphere or large ice cube in a rocks glass. —*DARREN*

 SERVES 1

---

2 ounces Vanilla Anise Whiskey

1 demerara sugar cube or 1 teaspoon brown sugar

Ice

3 dashes orange bitters

Generous swath of lemon zest, for garnish

1 Stir the infused whiskey and brown sugar in a shaker tin or mixing glass until the sugar dissolves. Add the ice and bitters. Stir gently for 20 turns to chill the drink. Strain into a coupe glass.

2 Twist the lemon swath over the drink to release its oils, rub on the rim of the glass, then drop into the cocktail.

Vanilla Anise Whiskey

12 ounces small batch rye whiskey

2 scored vanilla beans

2 pieces star anise

Seal in a Mason jar for 24 to 36 hours.

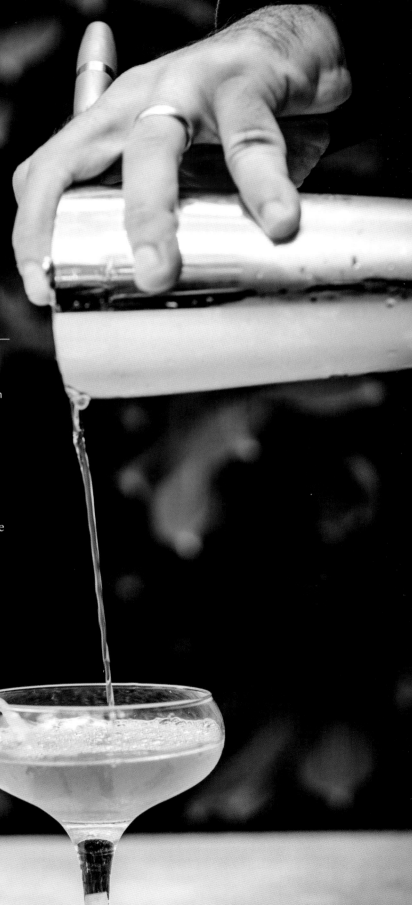

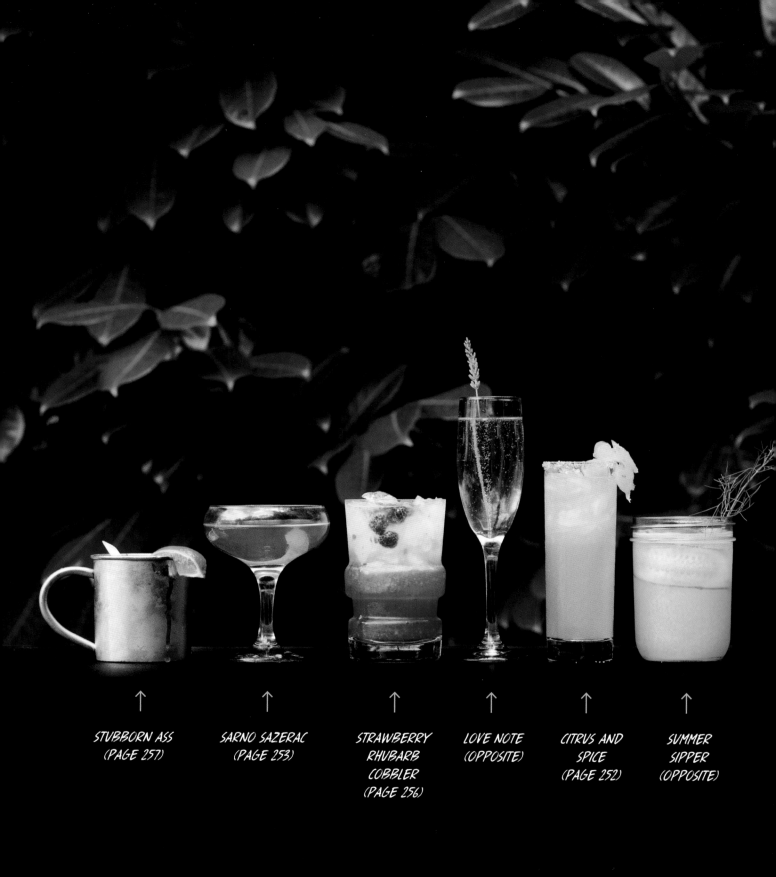

STUBBORN ASS
(PAGE 257)

SARNO SAZERAC
(PAGE 253)

STRAWBERRY
RHUBARB
COBBLER
(PAGE 256)

LOVE NOTE
(OPPOSITE)

CITRUS AND
SPICE
(PAGE 252)

SUMMER
SIPPER
(OPPOSITE)

SUMMER SIPPER

This drink has such a fresh, citrus nose, you want to stick your whole face in it before you take a sip. Hendrick's gin is popular in cucumber cocktails. Garnish this drink with a mint spring and a paper-thin cucumber ribbon. —*DARREN*

 SERVES 1

---

2 ounces Lime Gin

2 ounces Wicked Lemon Sour Mix

2 ounces fresh cucumber juice

Ice

Fresh lime wedge

Pour the infused gin, sour mix, and cucumber juice over ice in a shaker tin. Shake vigorously for 10 seconds. Strain over crushed ice in a Mason jar or pint glass. Squeeze in the juice from the lime wedge, then drop it into the drink.

Lime Gin

12 ounces small batch gin

4 large swaths of lime zest

Seal in a Mason jar for 24 to 36 hours.

Wicked Lemon Sour Mix

1 cup fresh lemon juice

1 cup agave syrup

Stir and chill for up to 1 day.

- For a nonalcoholic cocktail, combine the sour mix with ginger beer.

- For quick lemonade, mix with filtered water and crushed ice.

LOVE NOTE

Here's a sexy drink to serve in a classy champagne flute. Just a hint of lavender gives it a soothing aroma while the bubbles tickle your nose. —*DARREN*

 SERVES 1

½ ounce Lavender Vodka

¼ ounce grapefruit juice

⅛ ounce Lavender Syrup

4 ounces Prosecco

Pour the infused vodka, grapefruit juice, and lavender syrup in a flute (champagne) glass. Top with Prosecco.

Lavender Vodka

12 ounces vodka

1 sprig lavender flowers (½ tablespoon)

1 grapefruit swath

Seal in a Mason jar for 12 to 24 hours.

Lavender Syrup

← MIX WITH BUBBLY WATER FOR A LAVENDER SODA!

1 cup water

1 cup organic cane sugar

4 sprigs lavender flowers (2 tablespoons)

Simmer in a saucepot until the syrup thickens (8 to 10 minutes), then strain and cool.

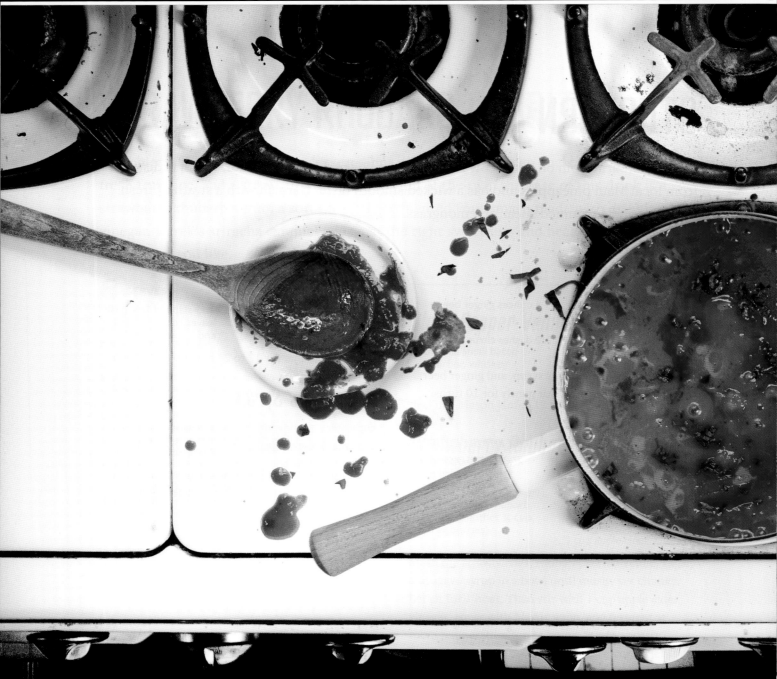

SAUCES AND BASICS

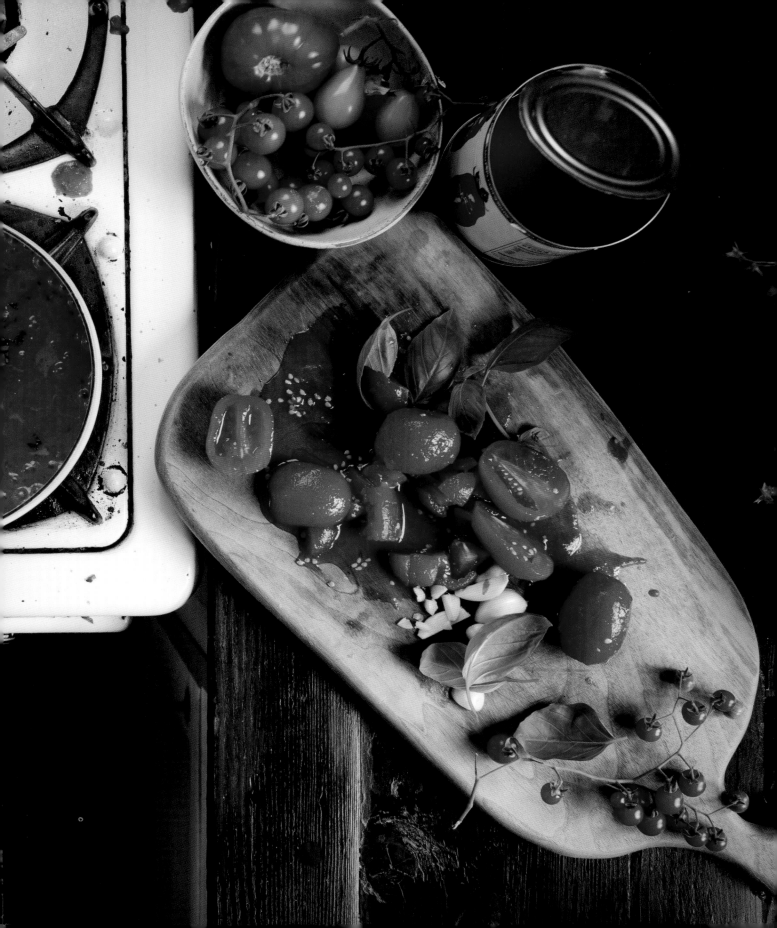

WICKED HEALTHY CHEESE SAUCE

This is one of those slam-dunk mother sauces. Don't let a couple of weird ingredients like nutritional yeast (or as I call it, hippy fish food) scare you. This is not hippy food. It just happens to be healthy. And it works with everything. At Whole Foods Market, I developed a version called Vegan Mac Sauce. Want it thicker? Add less soy milk. Want it like a Mexican queso sauce for nachos? Add Hatch chiles, cilantro, cumin, and chili powder. Instead of the squash, try it with different orange vegetables like carrots, sweet potatoes, or golden beets. You can take this recipe in any direction. You could even drop in some Thai chiles, Thai basil, and a squirt of lime to take it Eastward. Oh, and did we mention that it happens to be gluten-free, dairy-free, sugar-free, and oil-free? So much free! —*DEREK*

 MAKES ABOUT 1 QUART (1 HIGH-SPEED BLENDER LOAD)

1 cup raw cashews

2 cups chopped peeled butternut squash (frozen also works)

¼ cup garlic cloves (8 to 10 cloves), peeled

2 tablespoons rice vinegar

2 cups unsweetened soy milk

3 tablespoons nutritional yeast

2 tablespoons white miso (chickpea miso is an option)

2 teaspoons sea salt

1 teaspoon freshly ground black pepper

1 teaspoon smoked paprika

½ teaspoon ground white pepper

⅛ teaspoon cayenne pepper

1 Soak the cashews overnight in water to cover. Drain.

2 Combine the drained cashews, squash, garlic, and vinegar in a medium saucepot. Add water to cover (4 to 5 cups), and bring to a simmer over medium heat. Simmer until everything is super soft and smushable, 10 to 15 minutes.

3 Drain, and then pour the solid ingredients into a high-speed blender and start blending low and slow. Increase the speed, and gradually add the soy milk. When the milk is fully incorporated, add the remaining ingredients and blend on high until super smooth, 3 to 5 minutes. Like cream-sauce smooth. Use immediately or refrigerate for up to 1 week.

> **Pro Tip**
> *If you cook this sauce, it will thicken up. To adjust the consistency, add more or less soy milk (or other nondairy milk).*

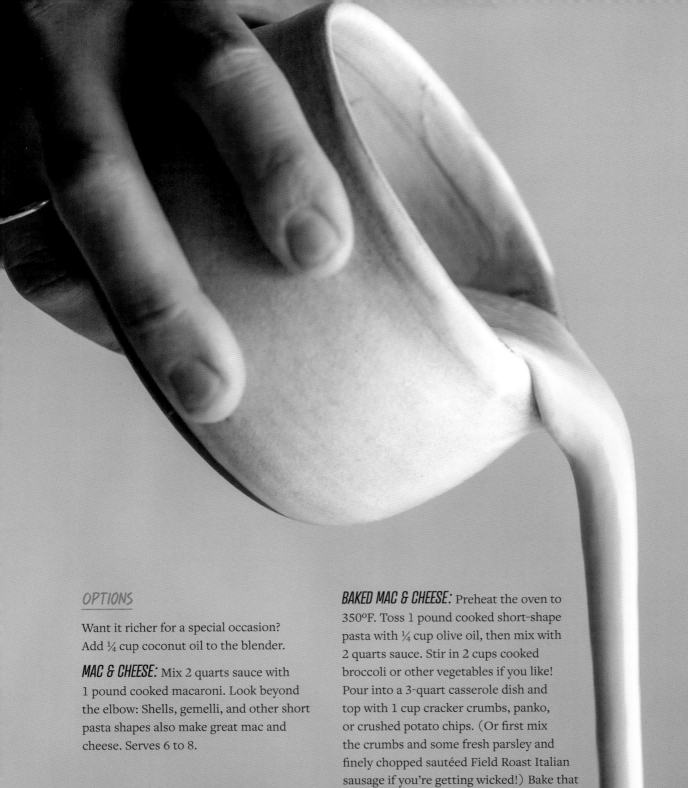

OPTIONS

Want it richer for a special occasion?
Add ¼ cup coconut oil to the blender.

MAC & CHEESE: Mix 2 quarts sauce with
1 pound cooked macaroni. Look beyond
the elbow: Shells, gemelli, and other short
pasta shapes also make great mac and
cheese. Serves 6 to 8.

BAKED MAC & CHEESE: Preheat the oven to
350°F. Toss 1 pound cooked short-shape
pasta with ¼ cup olive oil, then mix with
2 quarts sauce. Stir in 2 cups cooked
broccoli or other vegetables if you like!
Pour into a 3-quart casserole dish and
top with 1 cup cracker crumbs, panko,
or crushed potato chips. (Or first mix
the crumbs and some fresh parsley and
finely chopped sautéed Field Roast Italian
sausage if you're getting wicked!) Bake that
mac daddy until nicely browned on top,
about 30 minutes. Serves 6 to 8.

CAULIFLOWER MORNAY SAUCE

Mornay is a creamy French white sauce. Our plant-powered version gets its sexy texture from cooked and pureed cauliflower and cashews. Use this basic white sauce to add velvety richness to everything from steamed broccoli to pasta dishes, pizza, potatoes, and Spicy Maitake Steak Sandwiches (page 123).

 MAKES ABOUT 2 QUARTS

1½ cups raw cashews

1 head cauliflower, cut into large florets

4 to 5 cloves garlic, thinly sliced

1 bay leaf

2 tablespoons white miso

1 tablespoon sea salt

2 teaspoons freshly ground black pepper

3 cups unsweetened soy or almond milk

1 Soak the cashews in water to cover for 1 hour. Drain and rinse.

2 Transfer the rinsed cashews to a large saucepot. Add the raw cauliflower pieces, garlic, and bay leaf. Cover with water and bring to a simmer over medium heat. Simmer gently until the cauliflower is tender, 10 to 12 minutes. Drain and rinse, then remove and discard the bay leaf.

3 Transfer the solids to a blender (preferably high-speed). If you have a 2-quart blender, you can blend all the solids at once. For a 1-quart blender, do it in two batches. Add the miso, salt, and pepper and begin blending on low speed. Slowly add the soy milk, then increase the speed and blend until completely smooth, 3 to 5 minutes. Use immediately or cover and refrigerate for a few days. If it's too thick when reheated, add a little soy milk to thin it out.

MUSHROOM GRAVY TRAIN

Thick, creamy, and delicious—hop on the gravy train! Apply this gravy liberally to mashed potatoes, pan-seared mushrooms, or Smoky Poutine (page 72).

MAKES ABOUT 2 QUARTS

1 cup raw cashews

1 tablespoon plant-based butter

1 large onion, diced

1 tablespoon minced garlic

¼ cup dried mushroom powder (porcini, shiitake, etc.; see Pro Tips)

1 teaspoon poultry seasoning

½ teaspoon granulated onion

3 cups water

1 russet potato, peeled (or not; see Pro Tips) and rough chopped

½ teaspoon freshly ground black pepper

1 tablespoon fresh thyme leaves

1 tablespoon fresh rosemary leaves

¾ teaspoon sea salt

1 cup soy milk or other nondairy milk

1 Soak the cashews in water to cover overnight. Drain and rinse.

2 Heat a medium saucepan over medium heat. When hot, add the butter, diced onion, garlic, mushroom powder, poultry seasoning, and ¼ teaspoon of the granulated onion. Then add the drained cashews, water, potato, and black pepper. Bring the mixture to a simmer, then cut the heat to low and let simmer gently until the flavors blend, about 30 minutes.

3 Let cool a bit, then blend carefully in a blender (preferably high-speed), slowly at first, then gradually speeding up, until super smooth and sexy. Add the remaining ¼ teaspoon granulated onion and the thyme, rosemary, salt, and soy milk and blend it in. Taste the gravy and add more seasoning if you think it needs it. The gravy can be made a day or two ahead if you want. Just keep it in the fridge.

> **Pro Tips**
>
> → *Can't find mushroom powder? Make it! Buzz about ¾ cup dried mushrooms in a clean coffee grinder or spice mill to make about ¼ cup powder.*
>
> → *If you have a badass high-speed blender, you can just chop the potato without peeling it because the peel will get blitzed in the blender anyway. Like most vegetable peels, potato peels add healthy fiber to your diet.*

PLANT-BASED MAYO

Here's another staple recipe from our collaborator, David Joachim. It's simple, versatile, and totally wicked on sandwiches.

 MAKES ABOUT 1 CUP

¼ cup liquid from a can of chickpeas

THE CLOUDIER THE BETTER

1 tablespoon fresh lemon juice

1 teaspoon mustard powder

Dash cayenne pepper

Sea salt and freshly ground black pepper to taste

1 cup mild-flavored oil (a mix of grapeseed and olive oil is good)

1 Combine the chickpea liquid, lemon juice, mustard, cayenne, and a pinch each of salt and pepper in a blender (a stick blender also works well for this small amount). Blend briefly to combine.

2 With the blender running, add the oil in a slow trickle. Do not add it all at once. As the oil incorporates and the mixture thickens, increase the trickle to a slow, steady stream. Continue blending until all the oil is added and the mixture thickens. Taste and blend in additional seasonings as needed. Use immediately or refrigerate for up to 1 week.

OPTIONS

SRIRACHA MAYO: Stir in ⅓ cup Homemade Badass Sriracha (page 276) or Ninja Squirrel sriracha or other store-bought sriracha. Store in a squeeze bottle or empty sriracha bottle that has a squeeze top.

SRIRACHA RUSSIAN DRESSING: Mix ¾ cup mayo with ¼ cup finely chopped dill pickles, 2 tablespoons sriracha, 1½ tablespoons tomato paste, 1½ tablespoons finely chopped shallots, 1 tablespoon minced fresh parsley, 1 teaspoon Dijon mustard, ¼ teaspoon sea salt, and a grinding of freshly ground black pepper.

NANA SARNO'S RED SAUCE

Our nana was a second-generation Italian American who lived in Billerica, Massachusetts. Whenever you walked through her door, the aromas of this red sauce filled your nose with anticipation. Every time, no matter what time of day. She could be making meatballs, sausages, lasagna, or manicotti. Any way, this sauce was the gravy, the glue that held everything together—sometimes, it held the family together, too! It's a simple sauce, but you can't just throw everything in a pot. That would make a stew or a fresh pomodoro sauce. To make this classic, slow-simmered red sauce, you have to build layers of flavor one by one. Follow these steps and you'll always have a great sauce to hold together whatever dish you are making.

 MAKES 6 TO 8 CUPS

Everyday olive oil

1 white onion, diced small

2 large cloves garlic, minced

1 red bell pepper, diced small

1½ teaspoons minced fresh oregano

Sea salt and freshly ground black pepper

2 cans (28 ounces each) San Marzano tomatoes, drained

1 can (6 ounces) tomato paste

About ¼ teaspoon organic cane sugar, optional (see Pro Tips)

Large handful of basil leaves, torn

1 Heat a large saucepot over medium-high heat. Add enough oil to cover the bottom of the pot. Sauté the onions in the oil until they look golden around the edges, about 4 minutes. Add the garlic, bell pepper, and oregano. Sprinkle with a little salt and pepper, then sauté until the peppers are soft, about 5 minutes.

2 Use your hands to pinch and pull out the canned tomatoes' cores, then crush the tomatoes right into the pot. Add the tomato paste and sugar. Fill the tomato paste can 4 times with water, adding the water to the pan, and stir until incorporated. Simmer the sauce uncovered over low heat for 1 to 1½ hours, stirring now and then to prevent burning.

Use an immersion blender in the pot, or an upright blender, to puree the sauce—or, for the perfect rustic texture, use a food mill.

3 Return the sauce to low heat and simmer until the flavors blend, an additional 1 to 1½ hours. Taste the sauce, and add salt, pepper, and sugar until it tastes good to you. Remove from the heat and stir in the basil.

Pro Tips

→ *Cheater chopping: Pulse the onion in a food processor. While it's sautéing, pulse the garlic and bell pepper as well. Then chop the canned tomatoes the same way. If you use a food mill when it's done cooking, the mill will strain out the seeds for you.*

→ *Nana used fresh tomatoes whenever possible. To do that, peel, seed, and chop 6 pounds fresh San Marzano tomatoes and use instead of the canned.*

→ *If your tomatoes are sweet enough, you will not need the pinch of sugar. Alternatively, you could get a little sweetness by adding ½ cup finely shredded carrot when sautéing the onions.*

SMOKY BBQ SAUCE

Savory, smoky barbecue sauce has a slew of uses in plant-based cooking. Spread it on sandwiches instead of ketchup, or slather it on your favorite plants toward the end of grilling. Most BBQ sauces start with a base of ketchup, but we're not crazy about the corn syrup in ketchup. We use tomato paste as a base and build up the flavors from there.

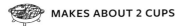 **MAKES ABOUT 2 CUPS**

2 tablespoons everyday olive oil

1 white onion, diced

4 cloves garlic, chopped

1 tablespoon smoked paprika

½ tablespoon ancho chile powder

1 teaspoon ground cumin

¾ cup tomato paste

1 chipotle in adobo sauce, finely chopped

1¼ cups Vegetable Stock (page 284) or store-bought

3 tablespoons red wine vinegar

3 tablespoons coconut sugar or brown sugar

2 tablespoons maple syrup

1½ tablespoons plant-based Worcestershire sauce

1 tablespoon grainy mustard

2 teaspoons sea salt

½ teaspoon freshly ground black pepper

1 Heat a large heavy-bottom pot over medium-high heat. Add the oil, then the onions and cook until nicely browned, 4 to 6 minutes, stirring now and then. Stir in the garlic and cook for about a minute.

2 Stir in the paprika, ancho powder, and cumin and let the spices toast with the onions for a minute or so, stirring once or twice. Stir in the tomato paste and chipotle to make a thick paste. Then stir in the remaining ingredients until everything is nice and smooth.

3 Cut the heat to medium low and simmer gently until the sauce reduces in volume by about one-fourth, about 8 minutes. If you like your sauce real thick, simmer it a little longer, stirring now and then to prevent burning on the bottom.

4 Remove from the heat and use immediately, or let cool and keep in a container in the fridge for up to a week or so.

NINJA TAMARI GLAZE

Math is hard. Playing with your food is not. Use this glaze like liquid flavor. And try mixing it up: Want some fresh herbs? Add a few basil or mint leaves. Into spices? Add a piece of star anise or a few cinnamon sticks or cardamom pods. Want more brightness? Squeeze in some fresh lemon or lime juice. Maybe stir in some tomato paste. Flavor it however you like. The mix all gets strained in the end anyway. Nail the basic mix and you're halfway to becoming an expert. Create a new flavor combo and you're the Yoda of your Dagobah. And how do you use it? Paint onto grilled or roasted vegetables or seared tofu. Mix into fried rice or vegetables. Brush it onto your best friend's naked body. Or thin it with a little water and make it a dip or drizzle for Summer Vegetable Carpaccio (page 191). —*DEREK*

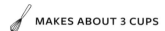 **MAKES ABOUT 3 CUPS**

2 cups water

1 cup low-sodium tamari

½ cup demerara sugar or light brown sugar

⅓ cup Ninja Squirrel sriracha, Homemade Badass Sriracha (page 276), or other sriracha

1 tablespoon rough chopped ginger

1 tablespoon rough chopped garlic

1 bay leaf

1 teaspoon arrowroot or cornstarch

2 tablespoons cold water

1 Combine the 2 cups water, tamari, sugar, sriracha, ginger, garlic, and bay leaf in a medium saucepot. Bring to a simmer over medium heat and simmer for about 5 minutes.

2 Whisk the arrowroot with the 2 tablespoons cold water (called a slurry), then whisk the slurry into the pot. Bring back to a simmer and simmer to cook out the starchy taste, 5 to 8 minutes. Shut off the heat and let sit for 5 minutes.

3 Strain the mixture through a fine-mesh strainer into a chillable container and let cool. Seal and refrigerate for up to 1 month.

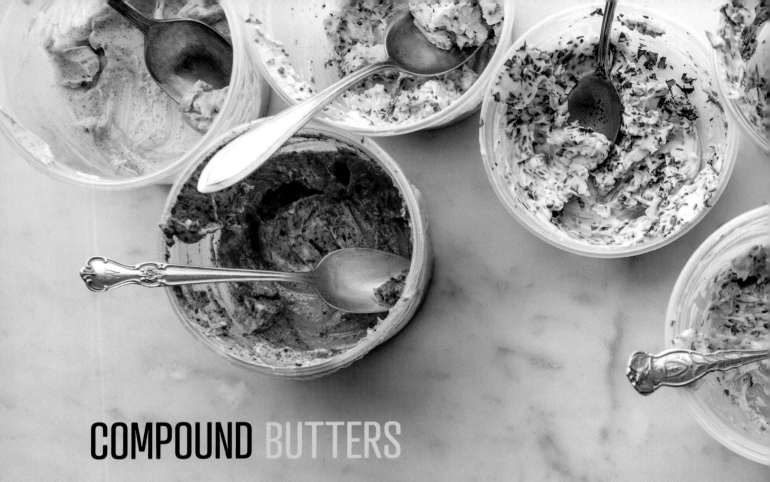

COMPOUND BUTTERS

The sky's the limit here. You like it spicy? Whip up some Sriracha Shallot Butter. Sweet's your thing? Try Apple Pie Butter or Strawberry Vanilla Butter. Maybe you like lots of aroma. Go for Tarragon Mustard Butter. Experiment with your favorite flavors—from herbs and spices to aromatics and sweeteners! You can spread compound butter on toast, use it to finish a sauce, or flavor a dessert with it. —CHAD

 MAKES ABOUT ½ CUP (1 STICK)

½ cup (1 stick) plant-based butter (such as Miyoko's or Earth Balance sticks)

1½ to 3 tablespoons flavoring (see the Options)

1 Mix the butter and flavoring in a food processor, in a stand mixer, or by hand. Use a food processor if you want to puree all the ingredients together and evenly color the butter. Mix by hand if you want to preserve chunks of flavoring/color in the butter. If mixing by hand or in a stand mixer, soften the butter at room temperature for 10 to 15 minutes while you prep the flavoring.

2 Once mixed, you can put the butter in a tub for scooping or shape it any way you like, then chill it. For pats, place the soft blended butter on parchment or plastic wrap, roll into a cylinder, and seal the ends. Keep chilled until ready to use.

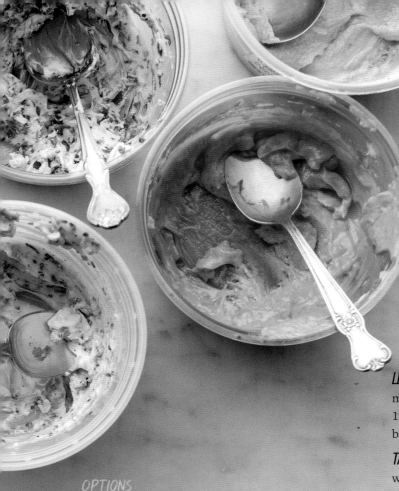

Spicy

SRIRACHA SHALLOT BUTTER: 2 tablespoons sriracha, 1 tablespoon minced shallot

JALAPEÑO, CILANTRO, AND LIME BUTTER: 1 tablespoon minced jalapeño, 1½ tablespoons minced fresh cilantro, 1 tablespoon lime juice, 1 teaspoon lime zest

HOT ROASTED PEPPER BUTTER: 2 tablespoons minced roasted red bell pepper, ½ tablespoon paprika, ½ teaspoon cayenne

Aromatic

ROASTED GARLIC AND PARSLEY BUTTER: 2 tablespoons roasted garlic paste (or 1½ tablespoons minced fresh garlic), 1 tablespoon granulated onion, 1 tablespoon minced fresh parsley

LEMON PEPPER CHIVE BUTTER: 1½ tablespoons minced fresh chives, ½ tablespoon minced shallot, 1 teaspoon lemon zest, ½ teaspoon freshly ground black pepper

TARRAGON MUSTARD BUTTER: 1 tablespoon coarse whole-grain mustard, ½ tablespoon minced fresh tarragon, ½ teaspoon minced shallots

UMAMI BUTTER: 1½ tablespoons ground dried shiitake mushrooms (buzzed in a spice mill), ½ tablespoon toasted sesame seeds, 1 teaspoon dark soy sauce

Sweet

VANILLA BUTTER: Seeds scraped from 1 split vanilla bean, 1½ tablespoons date sugar or maple sugar, ½ teaspoon vanilla extract

APPLE PIE BUTTER: 2 tablespoons minced dried apples, 1½ tablespoons maple sugar (or demerara sugar or brown sugar), 1 teaspoon cinnamon, ¼ teaspoon nutmeg, pinch of salt

STRAWBERRY VANILLA BUTTER: 2 tablespoons crushed freeze-dried strawberries, seeds scraped from ½ split vanilla bean, 1 teaspoon organic cane sugar

VAN DRUNEN FARMS MAKES GREAT FREEZE-DRIED FRUIT

HEIRLOOM TOMATO SALSA

We know people buy jarred salsa and "fresh" salsa in refrigerated plastic tubs. But it's soooo easy and so much better to mix up a fresh salsa at home. Use those oddly shaped multi-colored heirloom tomatoes from the farmers' market. —*DEREK*

 MAKES ABOUT 3 CUPS

2 large heirloom tomatoes, diced small

½ small red onion, diced small and rinsed

1–2 jalapeño peppers, seeded and diced small

LEAVE IN THE SEEDS IF YOU LIKE IT SPICY

1 lime, juiced

¼ cup chopped fresh cilantro

½ teaspoon sea salt

Lightly toss everything together in a medium serving bowl. Sometimes if the tomatoes are too juicy, we'll drain off some liquid.

POACHED CORN SALSA

We love tacos so much that we created a whole category of toppings called Taco Ticklers, page 112. Here's one of our favorite ticklers. Use it instead of your typical tomato-based salsa. It's perfect in late summer when sweet corn comes into the markets.

 MAKES ABOUT 3 CUPS

2 tablespoons plant-based butter

1 tablespoon sea salt

2 cups fresh corn kernels (from 3 to 5 ears sweet corn)

1 red jalapeño chile, seeded

1 cup diced baby cucumber (skin, seeds, and all)

¼ cup chopped fresh cilantro, plus a few leaves for garnish

1 lime, juiced

½ teaspoon freshly ground black pepper

1 Fill a medium saucepot with water (about 6 cups) and bring to a boil. Add the butter and 1½ teaspoons of the salt. Add the corn and return to a boil, then simmer for 1 minute. You're really just blanching or lightly poaching the kernels here instead of fully cooking them.

2 Drain the corn in a strainer, then let cool in the strainer. Do not rinse (you want that nice light coating of butter on the kernels).

3 Meanwhile, cut a few thin slices of jalapeño for garnish and set aside. Chop the rest of the jalapeño and transfer to a mixing bowl. Stir in the cooled corn, cucumber, cilantro, lime juice, the remaining 1½ teaspoons salt, and the pepper. Mix well. Chill for at least 1 hour or up to 1 day. Garnish with cilantro and jalapeño before serving.

HOMEMADE BADASS SRIRACHA

Personally, I can't stand the taste of ketchup. Since the '90s, I've been using sriracha instead. At Whole Foods Market, I developed a good, clean sriracha called Ninja Squirrel, named after my backyard pet, Zelda. It's a high-flavor, low-sodium, plant-based, and non-GMO sauce, and it's become a bestseller. According to *Time* magazine, even Hillary Clinton carries Ninja Squirrel sriracha in her bag while traveling! Here's the version I make at home. The key is keeping the green chile tops for a grassy, floral aroma in the final sauce. —*DEREK*

 MAKES ABOUT 4 CUPS

4½ pounds fresh Fresno or red jalapeño chiles, rinsed

20 medium cloves garlic, peeled

¾ cup molasses sugar or coconut sugar (see Pro Tips)

¼ cup sea salt

1¼ cups distilled white vinegar

1 Caution: Chile fumes burn! Strap a bandana around your face and don't touch the cut parts of the chiles. Or wear gloves when making this!

2 Use scissors to snip the stems from the chiles, but leave some of the green tops, which give the sriracha a grassy, floral aroma. Roughly chop the chiles and transfer to a food processor. Add the garlic, sugar, and salt and process until the mixture is pureed to the consistency of a smoothie, 30 seconds or so.

3 Pour the puree into a glass bowl or jar to ferment. I like glass so I can see the fermentation bubbles forming. You'll get a bit more fermentation from a large bowl or jar with a lot of airspace, instead of a bowl that barely fits the total volume of the puree. Cover with plastic wrap or a lid and let ferment at room temperature for 3 to 4 days. Uncover and stir about once a day. I like to use a rubber spatula to

make sure any bubble splatters get scraped from the inside of the bowl and mixed back into the puree, but that's not strictly necessary. If you've ever fermented anything, you know it will start to get funky smelling. Not bad funky, but good funky!

4 When lots of bubbles have formed, after about 4 days depending on the temperature in your kitchen, transfer the mixture to a high-speed blender and add the vinegar. Blend until it's as smooth as you can get it, 2 to 3 minutes. The seeds won't blend, but everything else should be pretty smooth.

5 Use a fine-mesh strainer and rubber spatula to press and strain the mixture through the strainer into a small saucepot. Place the pot of smooth puree over medium heat and bring it to a boil. Lower the heat so that the mixture simmers and simmer gently until the mixture reduces in volume by almost half, about 10 minutes. Open the windows because those chile fumes will get airborne! When the sauce is done, it should be thick enough to coat the back of a spoon. I like my sriracha a bit thick so I can squirt it without it splashing too much. If you like it thinner, just simmer it for less time.

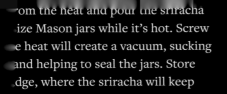

...om the heat and pour the sriracha ...ize Mason jars while it's hot. Screw ...e heat will create a vacuum, sucking ...and helping to seal the jars. Store ...dge, where the sriracha will keep

Pro Tips

→ *If you can't find molasses sugar or coconut sugar, you can use muscovado sugar or Barbados sugar. You can also use dark brown sugar, but the flavor won't be quite as floral.*

→ *Store some of this sriracha in an empty squeeze bottle (preferably one from an old bottle of sriracha), so you can squirt it onto sandwiches, bowls, rice, and whatever else at a moment's notice.*

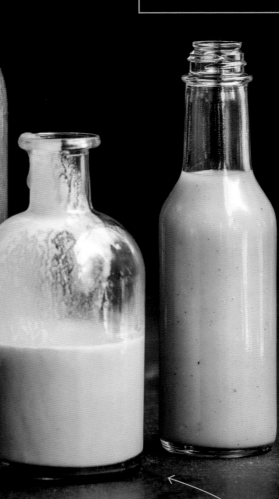

...EMADE BADASS SRIRACHA   CREAMY JALAPEÑO SALSA   CARROT HABANERO CITRUS HOT SAUCE

CARROT HABANERO CITRUS HOT SAUCE

Once or twice a year I get together with friends in Austin, Texas, for a hot sauce party. We harvest fresh chiles from our gardens, gather up gloves and bandanas, and spend the day making hot sauce, eating tacos, and drinking beer. A premium Sunday. Bonus: Everyone goes home with a few different flavors. This is one of my favorites. —CHAD

 MAKES 3 CUPS

Spray oil

1 large sweet white onion, chopped (about 1¼ cups)

3 cloves garlic, peeled

2 carrots, peeled and chopped

7 fresh habanero chile peppers, stemmed and seeded

LEAVE IN THE SEEDS IF YOU LIKE IT REALLY HOT!

1 cup fresh tangerine juice (from 4 to 6 tangerines)

½ lime, juiced

¾ cup distilled white vinegar

2 tablespoons organic cane sugar

2 tablespoons sea salt

1½ teaspoons lemon zest, optional

1 Preheat the oven to 450°F.

2 Coat a baking sheet with spray oil and spread the onions in a single layer on the pan. Roast until the onions are slightly charred, 10 to 12 minutes. Even just a little charring adds a ton of flavor to the sauce.

3 Meanwhile, heat a small heavy skillet (we like cast iron) over medium heat. Add the garlic cloves and cook until the garlic blackens in spots, 4 to 5 minutes, shaking the pan occasionally. Again, the blackening is flavor.

4 Transfer the onions and garlic to a large pot along with the carrots, habaneros, tangerine juice, lime juice, vinegar, sugar, salt, and lemon zest (if using). Bring to a boil over high heat, then lower the heat so the mixture simmers. Simmer until the sauce reduces in volume by about a third, 45 to 50 minutes. It should boil down quite a bit.

5 Use an immersion blender or upright blender to blend the mixture until it's pretty smooth. Return to the heat and simmer over medium heat until the sauce is thick enough to coat the back of a spoon, about 10 minutes. You want it thinner than ketchup but thicker than something like Worcestershire sauce. Keep simmering until you get that medium-thick hot sauce consistency.

6 Pour the sauce into two pint-size Mason jars while the sauce is hot. Screw on the lids. The heat will create a vacuum, sucking down the lids and helping to seal the jars. Store in the fridge. It'll keep for a month or so.

QUICK PICKLED VEGETABLES

I've been a fan of Andy Ricker's authentic Thai food for years. After moving to Portland, Oregon, I became even more enamored of him as a chef. Andy recently came out with a line of drinking vinegars that I can't get enough of. The intense concentrated flavors make food taste amazing. If you can't find Andy's Pok Pok Som Chinese celery drinking vinegar, called for here, replace it with ½ cup rice vinegar, 2 teaspoons sugar, and ½ teaspoon celery salt. Either way, you'll get some amazing pickles to serve with rice or sandwiches, or just to have as a snack.—*DEREK*

 MAKES TWO PINT-SIZE JARS

1 cup rice vinegar

½ cup Pok Pok Som Chinese celery drinking vinegar

¼ cup water

3 tablespoons organic cane sugar

½ red onion, cut into ½-inch-wide strips

1 small zucchini, cut into ¼-inch-thick rounds

1 medium carrot, cut on a diagonal into ¼-inch-thick ovals

1 jalapeño chile, cut into ¼-inch-thick rounds

4 cloves garlic, sliced

4 whole red Thai chiles

4 sprigs fresh oregano

½ teaspoon black peppercorns

1 In a medium bowl, whisk together the rice vinegar, drinking vinegar, water, and sugar until the sugar dissolves.

2 Divide everything else between two pint-size Mason jars or sealable containers. Pour the vinegar mixture evenly between both jars.

3 Refrigerate the jars overnight, and the pickles will be ready to use the next day. You can keep them in the fridge for several weeks. The longer they sit, the stronger and more vinegary the pickles will get.

PRESERVED MEYER LEMONS

This is one of those recipes that teaches patience. It takes very little handwork, but 3 weeks for the lemons to "cure" in the fridge. When they're done, the preserved lemons can be chopped and added to couscous, rice, pasta dishes, stews, sauces, salad dressings...almost anywhere you want a shot of salty-sour-sweet flavor. If your dish has already been salted, rinse off the excess salt before using the lemons. —*CHAD*

 MAKES ONE ½-GALLON JAR

REGULAR EUREKA
LEMONS ALSO WORK

9 to 12 Meyer lemons, scrubbed well

About 1 cup coarse sea salt

About ½ cup fresh squeezed Meyer lemon juice (from about 2 Meyer lemons)

1 Prepare the lemons one at a time: Cut off the green tip of the lemon. Then begin as if you were cutting the lemon in half lengthwise, but only let the knife go halfway down through the lemon. You're really slitting the lemon halfway through lengthwise. Turn the lemon about a quarter turn and make another slit halfway through. Repeat the process until you have 4 to 6 lengthwise slits all around the lemon. Repeat with the remaining lemons.

2 Next, open up each slit with your fingers and fill with a generous amount of salt, packing it in with your fingertips. Repeat with all the slits in all the lemons, stuffing each slit with salt. It may seem odd to use so much salt, but trust me. This is what makes the magic lemon pickles happen.

3 Next, stuff the lemons in a half-gallon glass jar (or two 1-quart jars). Squish them down so that some juice is squeezed from every lemon. Once all the lemons are stuffed in, sprinkle the remaining salt over them all; if you've already used all the salt for stuffing, sprinkle with about 2 tablespoons more salt.

Press the lemons again to ensure they are packed tight. There should be enough extracted lemon juice for the lemons to be covered in liquid, but if they are not completely covered, add enough fresh squeezed lemon juice to completely cover them.

4 Seal the jar tightly and let sit at room temperature for 3 or 4 days. About once a day, turn and gently shake the jar to redistribute the salt and spices (see the Option). After 3 or 4 days, place the jar in the fridge and chill for at least 3 weeks, again turning the jar every few days. After 3 weeks, the lemon rinds should be very soft. Have patience. It's a long process, but it's well worth the wait. Plus, preserved lemons keep in the fridge for at least 6 months.

5 When you want to use a preserved lemon, remove it from the jar and rinse it thoroughly but gently to remove excess salt and the seeds.

OPTION

• To spice it up, add 4 cinnamon sticks, 3 dried cayenne-type chiles, 2 tablespoons coriander seeds, and/or 1 tablespoon black peppercorns to the jar before you add the salt and lemons.

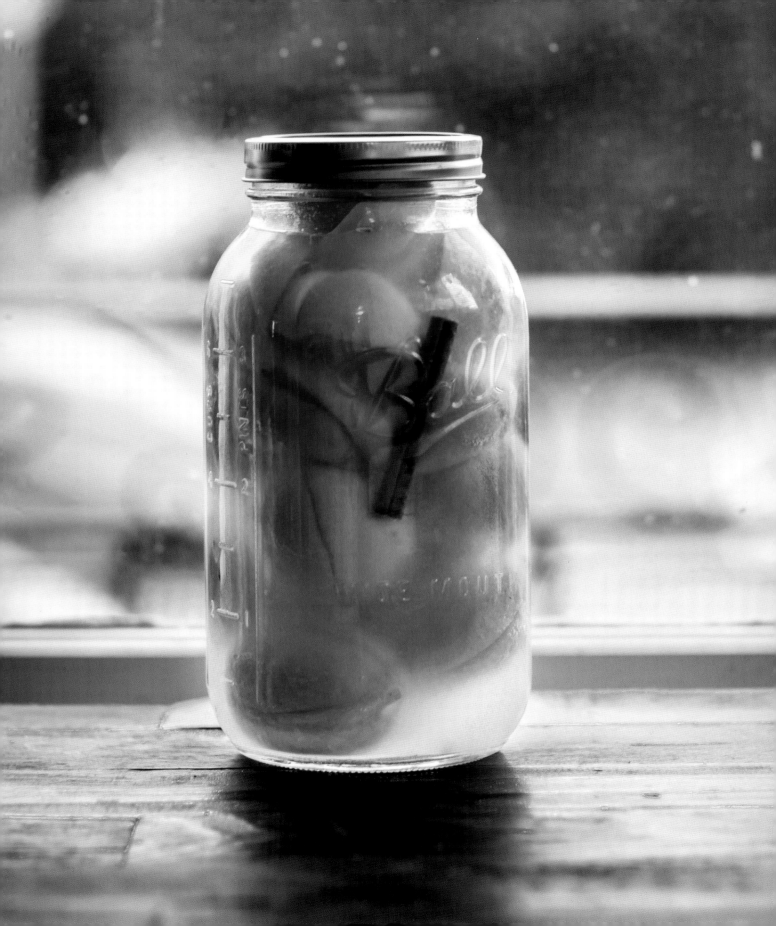

TOMATO HABANERO JAM

A good chutney tastes so spicy that you can barely eat it, but so sweet that you want to keep eating it anyway. That's what I was going for in this jam. When I first moved to Austin, Texas—a mecca for chileheads if I ever saw one—I started making a pineapple habanero jam with caramelized onions, lemon zest, and fresh thyme. It was good, but I wanted to put an Italian spin on it, so I tried it with tomatoes instead of pineapple. That came out even better. —*CHAD*

 MAKES ABOUT 2 CUPS

10 vine-ripened tomatoes, about 4 pounds

2 tablespoons everyday olive oil

1 sweet white onion, diced small (about 1½ cups)

6 cloves garlic, sliced wicked thin

6 to 10 habanero chile peppers, sliced or minced *WEAR GLOVES!*

2 cups organic cane sugar

3 tablespoons cider vinegar

1 tablespoon grated lemon zest

2 teaspoons minced fresh thyme

½ tablespoon sea salt

Pinch of ground white pepper

1 Bring a large pot of water to a boil. Set up a bowl of ice water.

2 Cut an X in the bottom of each tomato, then drop them into the boiling water and blanch until the skins start to peel back, about 30 seconds. Use a spider strainer or slotted spoon to transfer the tomatoes to the ice water. When cool, peel the skins from the tomatoes with your fingertips and a paring knife. Remove the cores and roughly chop the peeled tomatoes. You should have about 8 cups.

3 Heat the oil in a medium saucepan over low heat. Add the onions and sweat until soft, about 5 minutes. You don't want to brown the onions, just soften or "sweat" them. Add the garlic and continue sweating for 3 to 4 minutes more.

4 Add the chopped tomatoes and everything else and crank the heat to high. Bring the mixture to a simmer, then cut the heat to low. Let everything simmer gently until thickened to a soft jam-like consistency, 1 to 1¼ hours. With all that sugar, the jam will want to burn on the bottom. Don't let it. Stir the pot often to keep the jam from sticking and burning. The finished consistency should be like thin jam. It will thicken up more when it cools.

5 When the hot jam is nice and thick but still pourable, ladle or pour the jam into a pint-size Mason jar. Screw on the lid and let the jam sit at room temperature until cooled, 1 to 2 hours. The heat in the jar should create a vacuum, sucking down the lid. When cooled, store the jam in the fridge. It will keep for a few weeks.

COCONUT CORN BROTH

WE DON'T RECOMMEND THAT!

As New England boys, we have to say that organic, local corn tops the list of our most craved summertime foods. We have fond memories of throwing freshly gnawed corncobs at each other. How did coconut get into the picture? From Andy Ricker, the brilliant chef at Pok Pok in Portland, Oregon. Andy serves a grilled coconut corn on the cob during the summer, and it made me think of Thai soup, so I made a broth with some of those Thai flavors I love so much. Sweet, sour, spicy, salty, minty, gingery, garlicky...this broth's got it going on! —*DEREK*

 MAKES ABOUT 2 QUARTS

6 large ears corn, preferably organic and in season, shucked

3 quarts water

1 can (14 ounces) coconut milk or coconut cream

1 jalapeño chile, halved lengthwise (remove the seeds for less heat)

¼ cup thinly sliced fresh ginger

¼ cup garlic cloves (8 to 12 cloves), crushed with the flat of your knife

10 fresh mint sprigs, stems and all

1 bay leaf

1 star anise, optional

1 teaspoon sea salt

½ teaspoon ground white pepper

1 lime, juiced

1 Snap or cut the ears of corn in half.

2 Bring the water to a boil in a large stockpot over high heat. Add the corn and everything else except the lime juice. Cut the heat to medium, then bring the liquid to a slow simmer. Let it simmer for 10 to 15 minutes.

3 Remove the corncobs and cut the kernels from the cobs (see Pro Tips). Return the naked cobs to the broth along with the lime juice. Continue simmering gently over medium heat for another 30 minutes. The liquid will reduce in volume by about one-fourth, which is fine. Shut off the heat and let everything cool down a bit in the pot. Strain the warm broth through a fine-mesh strainer into quart containers, then use immediately or refrigerate for a week or two before using.

Pro Tips

→ *When the corn on the cob is tender, after 10 to 15 minutes of simmering, you could just take the cobs out of the broth and gnaw the corn off the cobs. But you want the naked cobs to go back in the broth for more flavor. So...if it's all in the family and you don't mind re-using the gnawed-down cobs, give them a quick rinse, then add them back to the broth. Or simply cut the tender kernels from the cobs as directed and serve the corn as loose kernels. You'll get about 5 cups corn kernels. You can keep them in the fridge for a few days or cool completely and freeze them for several weeks.*

→ *Use the corn kernels to make Poached Corn Salsa (page 275), Corn Dumplings in Coconut Corn Broth (page 87), or Spicy Coconut–Corn Crack (page 158).*

VEGETABLE STOCK

Every good soup starts with a great stock. A couple of keys to making one: First, taste the stock periodically as you make it, and only add additional salt and seasonings toward the end, because as the stock reduces in volume the flavors will concentrate. Second, we like to add potatoes to our vegetable stocks. The starches add body and give the stock a more satisfying consistency.

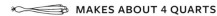 **MAKES ABOUT 4 QUARTS**

1½ gallons cold water

3 large carrots, scrubbed and rough chopped

1 large onion, peeled and quartered

1 leek, cleaned and rough chopped

4 stalks celery, rough chopped

1 large sweet potato (skin-on), scrubbed, cut in half

1 russet potato (skin-on), scrubbed, cut in half

1 fennel bulb, cleaned and rough chopped

¼ cup garlic cloves (8 to 12 cloves), peeled and crushed with the flat side of your knife

1 tablespoon black peppercorns

2 bay leaves

1 bunch parsley, rinsed

1 small bunch fresh thyme, rinsed

2 to 3 tablespoons sea salt

1 Put everything but the salt in a large stock pot. Bring to a slow simmer over medium heat, then cut the heat to low and simmer gently for a couple of hours. The more you simmer the stock, the more it will reduce in volume, and the more intense the flavors will become. Shoot to reduce the liquid by about one-half. A good visual is to simmer until the volume of stock is about 3 inches below the level it started at. When reduced and flavorful, add salt until it tastes well-seasoned to you.

2 Cool in the pot, then strain the stock into containers. Seal and refrigerate for about a week, or freeze for a couple of months.

OPTIONS

SPICY TOMATO VEGETABLE STOCK: Add a couple of Thai chiles and some chopped fresh tomato or a roasted tomato.

ROASTED VEGETABLE STOCK: Roast or grill all the vegetables or even just the onions and celery ahead of time. Get them slightly charred for a more robust flavor.

DARK VEGETABLE STOCK: Rub the carrots, onions, and celery with tomato paste and roast at 350°F for 1 hour before adding to the stock.

MUSHROOM STOCK: Skip the sweet potato and fennel. Instead, add 1 pound fresh cremini mushrooms and 5 ounces dried shiitake mushrooms (or use a mix of different fresh and dried 'shrooms). For more flavor, roast the fresh mushrooms first. For even more savory flavor, add ½ ounce dried seaweed such as kombu.

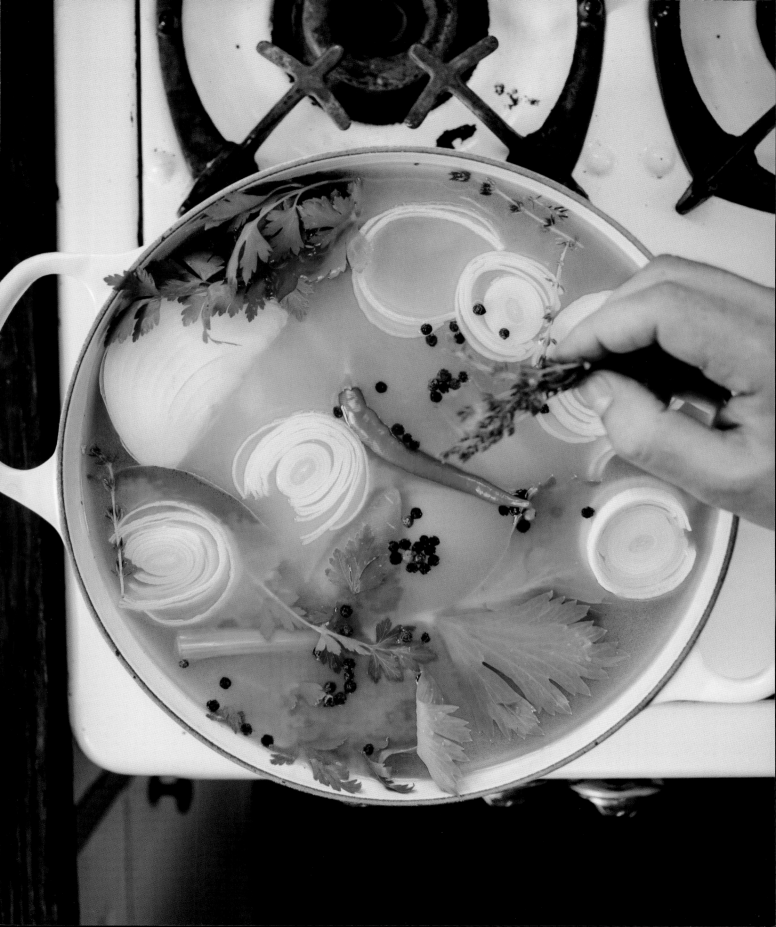

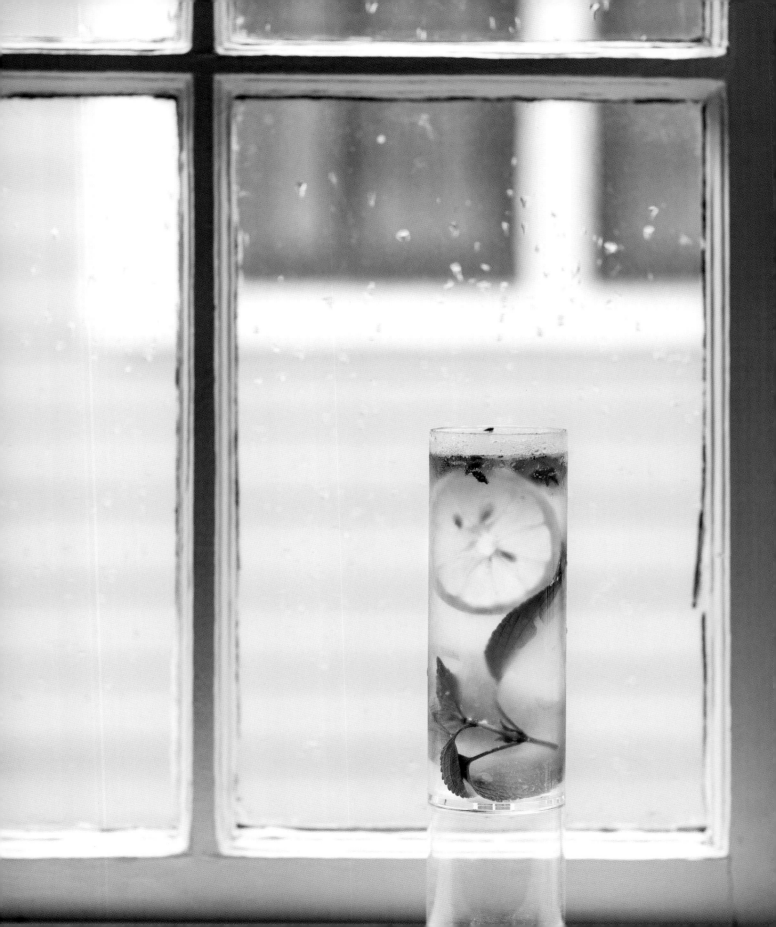

APPENDIX: *WICKED HEALTHY BENDERS AND SPECIAL DIETS*

A Wicked Healthy bender is like the opposite of binge eating. It's a cleanse. It's what you do to *recover* from bingeing. It's going on a bender of healthy eating to rejuvenate and recharge your system. Here are some ideas to get you started.

HIT-THE-RESET-BUTTON BENDER

A combination of juicing and light broths will kick-start your New Year's resolutions, or try these recipes any time of year you need to get back on track.

Cucumber, Celery, Green Apple, and Kale Juice—248

Spicy Pineapple, Spinach, Kale, and Lime Juice—248

Iron Man Juice—248

Vegetable Stock—284

Mushroom Stock—284

Coconut Corn Broth—283

RAW(ISH) BENDER

A selection of raw recipes in the book. They can also be garnished with some cooked components.

Nori Sunflower Snacks—55

Cashew au Poivre Torte with Basil Parsley Pesto—74

Summer Vegetable Carpaccio—191

Kale and Avocado Salad with Wild Rice, Grapes, and Toasted Seeds—199

Drunken Berries with Amaretto Gelato—230

Meyer Lemon Cheesecake with Grilled Peaches and Lavender Syrup—239

Wicked Healthy Juices (any)—248

WHOLE-FOOD BENDER

Just a few of the dishes in this book that are 100% whole foods with no processed ingredients, added sugars, or oils, and minimal sodium.

Nori Sunflower Snacks—55

Avocado Toasts with Radishes and Meyer Lemon (using whole-grain bread)—58

Slow-Cooked Corona Beans with Rosemary and Lots of Garlic—150

Potato and Cauliflower Bisque—157

Split Pea and Chard Soup—161

Four-Bean and Sweet Potato Slow-Cooker Chili—166

Kale Queso—176

Sweet Potato Gratin with Crispy Onions and Rosemary—185

GLUTEN-FREE DIET

If tamari or soy sauce is called for in any recipe, use wheat-free tamari. If any flour, bread, or bread crumbs are called for, choose a gluten-free option.

Ninja Nuts—52

Black Garlic and Chive Panisse with Citrus Aioli—53

Nori Sunflower Snacks—55

Grilled Sweet Potato, Sriracha Caramel, and Kale Toasts—56

Avocado Toasts with Radishes and Meyer Lemon—58

Minted Pea Ricotta, Grilled Zucchini, and Charred Lemon Toasts—60

Grilled Baby Artichoke Crostini with Cashew Crème Fraîche and Horseradish—61

Fiery Black Bean Spread—62

Minted Pea Ricotta—64

Toasted-Onion Sour Cream—65

Roasted Carrot-Lentil Dip—65

Wicked-Good Caponata—66

Tomato Confit—67

King Satay with Spicy Peanut-Ginger Sauce—70

Chickpea Blintzes with Cashew Sour Cream, Apples, and Dill—76

King Oyster Scallops with Shaved Asparagus and Corona Butter—79

Lion's Mane Steaks—90

Fresh Corn Tortillas—104

Hot Chocolate Lentil and Grilled Asparagus Tacos—108

Lion's Mane Street Tacos—110

Jackfruit Carnitas Tacos—114

Buddha Bowl—140

Banana Blossoms with Coconut and Chile—142

Bibimbap with Bamboo Rice—146

Slow-Cooked Corona Beans with Rosemary and Lots of Garlic—150

Stir-Fried Farro Fawcett—152

Forest Miso Soup—155

Spicy Coconut-Corn Crack—158

Split Pea and Chard Soup—161

Lobstah Mushroom Chowdah—162

Roasted Cauliflower Fagioli—164

Four-Bean and Sweet Potato Slow-Cooker Chili—166

NO-ADDED-SUGAR DIET

Sugar seems to be *everywhere* in today's food products. One of the best things about preparing your own food is that you can choose what types of sugars you use or eliminate them altogether. The recipes here do not use refined granulated or liquid sweeteners. Some of these recipes do include fresh fruits, dried fruits, and fruit pastes.

Black Garlic and Chive Panisse with Citrus Aioli—53

Avocado Toasts with Radishes and Meyer Lemon—58

Minted Pea Ricotta, Grilled Zucchini, and Charred Lemon Toasts—60

Minted Pea Ricotta—64

Roasted Carrot–Lentil Dip—65

Tomato Confit—67

Ma's Baked Spring Rolls—68

Smoky Poutine—72

Cashew au Poivre Torte with Basil Parsley Pesto—74

Chickpea Blintzes with Cashew Sour Cream, Apples, and Dill—76

King Oyster Scallops with Shaved Asparagus and Corona Butter—79

Corn Dumplings in Coconut Corn Broth—87

Lion's Mane Steaks—90

Sourdough Pizza Dough—96

Margherita Pizza—99

Fresh Corn Tortillas—104

Buddha Bowl—140

Banana Blossoms with Coconut and Chile—142

Slow-Cooked Corona Beans with Rosemary and Lots of Garlic—150

Forest Miso Soup—155

Potato and Cauliflower Bisque—157

Spicy Coconut–Corn Crack—158

Split Pea and Chard Soup—161

Lobstah Mushroom Chowdah—162

Roasted Cauliflower Fagioli—164

Oatmeal Bar—167

Painted Dijon Potatoes—175

Kale Queso—176

Whole Roasted Zucchini with Nana's Red Sauce—180

Baby Bok Choy with Roasted Kohlrabi Vinaigrette—181

Brussels Nachos—182

Sweet Potato Gratin with Crispy Onions and Rosemary—185

Smoky Cheesy Roasted Cauliflower Head—186

Summer Vegetable Carpaccio—191

Roasted Beet Salad with Citrus and Tarragon Cashew Cream—193

Kale and Avocado Salad with Wild Rice, Grapes, and Toasted Seeds—199

Spaghetti with Nana's Red Sauce—202

Cacio e Pepe with Lemon Chive Butter and Pink Peppercorns—204

Orecchiette with Grilled Squash, Preserved Lemon, and Herbs—205

Strozzapreti with Cauliflower Mornay, Mushrooms, and Kale—206

Pasta Dough—208

Porcini Ravioli with Garlic Butter and Sorrel—211

Spring Agnolotti with Favas, Mint, and Sherry Cream—214

Pumpkin Risotto with Chestnuts and Horseradish—216

Mac & Cheese Bar—218

Loaded Baked Potato Bar—220

Cucumber, Celery, Green Apple, and Kale Juice—248

Spicy Pineapple, Spinach, Kale, and Lime Juice—248

Iron Man Juice—248

Wicked Healthy Cheese Sauce—260

Cauliflower Mornay Sauce—262

Mushroom Gravy Train—263

Plant-Based Mayo—264

Nana Sarno's Red Sauce (omit sugar)—265

Compound Butters—268

Meme's Dressing—271

Carrot Coconut Dressing—272

Creamy Jalapeño Salsa—273

Heirloom Tomato Salsa—274

Poached Corn Salsa—275

Coconut Corn Broth—283

Vegetable Stock—284

NUT-FREE DIET

Nut allergies are a serious dietary restriction. The following recipes do not contain nuts or nut products. Some of these recipes may contain seeds, seed oils, and coconut. If peanut oil is called for, use another high-heat cooking oil such as grapeseed oil or sunflower oil. If the recipe calls for nut milk, choose soy, oat, hemp, or your favorite nut-free nondairy milk.

Black Garlic and Chive Panisse with Citrus Aioli—53

Nori Sunflower Snacks—55

Avocado Toasts with Radishes and Meyer Lemon—58

Minted Pea Ricotta—64

Roasted Carrot–Lentil Dip—65

Tomato Confit—67

Ma's Baked Spring Rolls—68

King Oyster Scallops with Shaved Asparagus and Corona Butter—79

Smoked Tofu Dumplings with Spinach, Dates, and Black Vinaigrette—84

Lion's Mane Steaks—90

Sourdough Pizza Dough—96

Fresh Corn Tortillas—104

Hot Chocolate Lentil and Grilled Asparagus Tacos—108

Lion's Mane Street Tacos—110

Jackfruit Carnitas Tacos—114

Samurai Burger with Wasabi, Sesame, Cucumber, and Kimchi Mayo—116

Sloppy BBQ Jackfruit Sliders with Slaw, Sriracha Mayo, and Pickles—118

New England Lobster Roll—120

Spicy Maitake Steak Sandwich—123

Banh Mi with Lemongrass Tofu and Ginger Aioli—124

PBLT—Plant-Based BLT with Tomato Habanero Jam and Herb Aioli—126

Plant Bacon—128

Kickass Plant-Based Reuben on Dark Rye (seitan pastrami and smoky beet versions)—133

Buddha Bowl (omit nuts from bowl)—140

Banana Blossoms with Coconut and Chile—142

Bibimbap with Bamboo Rice—146

Slow-Cooked Corona Beans with Rosemary and Lots of Garlic—150

Stir-Fried Farro Fawcett—152

Forest Miso Soup—155

SOY-FREE DIET

Soy is a megacrop that shows up in lots of food products. If you're avoiding soy, here are the recipes for you. For any recipe that calls for soy milk, swap in any other nondairy milk; choose soy-free plant-based butter when called for; and use Bragg liquid aminos instead of tamari or soy sauce.

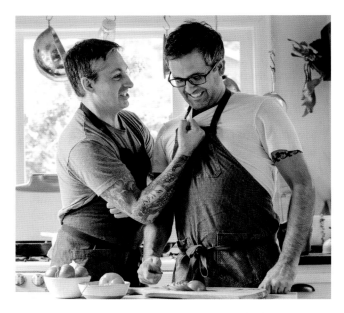

Ingredients

We love to simplify healthy cooking, and most of the ingredients in our recipes are widely available in grocery stores and health food stores. If you come across an ingredient that you can't find in a nearby market, surf the web. You can buy a slew of healthy foods and international foods, like vegan fish sauce, online. For hard-to-find American foods, go to panzers.co.uk. For Asian, try orientalmarket.co.uk, and for Mexican, visit mexgrocer.co.uk. We also provide lots of ingredient substitutions right in the recipes. As for ingredient names, we grew up in Boston, so we use American food terms. You are probably aware of most of these, given the cultural crossover between the UK and the US. Here are the ones we use most often: arugula is rocket, cilantro is fresh coriander, scallions are spring onions, snow peas are mangetout, zucchini are courgettes, squash are marrow, and eggplants are aubergines.

Measurements and Temperatures

Since we grew up in America, our recipes use teaspoon, tablespoon, and cup measurements for volume. Weights are listed in imperial ounces and pounds instead of metric milligrams and grams. Oven temperatures are given in degrees Fahrenheit instead of Celsius and gas marks. All of the conversions for UK kitchens are pretty simple. Just have a look at the charts.

Volume Equivalents

US measurements	Imperial equivalent	Metric equivalent
1 tsp	0.15 fl oz	5 mL
1 tbsp	0.5 fl oz	15 mL
2 tbsp	1 fl oz	25 mL
3 tbsp	1.5 fl oz	45 mL
¼ cup	2 fl oz	50 mL
⅓ cup	3 fl oz	75 mL
½ cup	4 fl oz	125 mL
⅔ cup	5 fl oz	150 mL
¾ cup	6 fl oz	175 mL
1 cup	8 fl oz	250 mL

Weight Equivalents

1 oz	30 g
2 oz	60 g
3 oz	90 g
4 oz	125 g
8 oz	250 g
10 oz	300 g
12 oz	375 g
1 lb	500 g
2 lbs	1 kg

Oven Temperature Equivalents

Degrees Fahrenheit (°F)	Degrees Celsius (°C)	Gas mark
225	110	¼
250	130	½
275	140	1
300	150	2
325	160	3
350	180	4
375	190	5
400	200	6
425	220	7
450	230	8
475	240	9

THANKS

What an incredible journey this book has been. We are grateful to everyone who helped it see the light of day, especially:

MY WIFE, MALISSA, FOR HER INFINITE PATIENCE, LOVE, AND SUPPORT; AND MY SWEET AMAYA AND LITTLE KAI FOR MOTIVATING ME TO MAKE THIS WORLD A LITTLE BIT BETTER
—CHAD

MY WICKED-AMAZING SON, JAKE; AMANDA AND THE WARDS, WHOSE LOVE MADE ME THE PERSON I AM TODAY; THE LOVELY MILDRED (MY FOSTER SQUIRREL) AND HANK, HER BROTHER; AND BUDDY THE FOX, MY HOUSEMATE IN LONDON
—DEREK

Dave Joachim, for all his amazing work and skill in dealing with two crazy brothers—and doing it with style.

Sally Ekus, our not-so-secret agent.

Our brother, Darren, for the killer cocktail recipes in the book and for huge support!

Our dad and Toni for their encouragement; and our extended family, including Nana, who inspired us both in the kitchen with her life-changing red sauce.

The whole team at Grand Central, including Sarah Pelz and Karen Murgolo for taking us on, Morgan Hedden for taking over, and the rest of the team for taking this book to the next level.

Toni Tajima for handling this book's many design challenges with aplomb.

Tal Ronnen for sharing a fantastic pasta dough recipe and smart tips about making pasta.

Sean Coyne for the insights into sourdough starters and the incredible pizza dough recipe.

Woody Harrelson for the foreword.

Eva Kosmas Flores, our wicked badass photographer, for the awesome images in the book, and food and prop stylist Sasha Swerdloff.

Khenpo, Khenchen, and all our friends at Padma Samye Ling for helping to clarify what compassionate action looks like.

Tucker Hall, Zach, and Josh for rooting for us the entire time.

Spring Water Farms, Smithy Farms, and all the mushroom growers and foragers out there.

The ones who paved the way with plant-based nutrition and served as a wake-up call to so many—thank you, Joel Fuhrman, MD; Caldwell Esselstyn, MD; Neal Barnard, MD; Michael Klaper, MD; Scott Stoll, MD; Rip Esselstyn; Margaret Wittenberg; and John Mackey.

Chris Kerr, Erin Wysocarski, Hiram Camillo Rodriquez, and the rest of the tribe that helped to get us on the map and continues to help Wicked Healthy grow.

All the plant pushers and the Wicked Healthy community for sharing the truth about eating plants and living with compassion.

Our intrepid crew of recipe testers, including Beverly Burl, Patti Oneil, Jess Kolko, Lisa Rice, Leanne Valenti, Josh Rininger, Dan Marek, Brian Stafford, Barb Thomas, Lauren Lewis, Jason Stefanko, Lydia Sadoudi, Adam Michaelson, Anna Franceschi, John Philips, Lisa Spudic Cusano, Marc Grika, Laura Price, Christina Martin, Beth Leonard, Michelle McNeal Daly, Debbie Deisher, Brianna Gallo, Yvette Schindler, Kerry Abdow, Kelly McShane.

All our friends and family whom we have neglected to mention by name, you know who you are and our hearts go out to you.

INDEX

Note: *Italic* page numbers refer to illustrations.

ABOUT THE AUTHORS

WICKED HEALTHY Founded by Derek Sarno and Chad Sarno, this thriving online community of plant pushers has quickly become the hub for sharing recipes and culinary inspiration. Wicked Healthy has been instrumental in the development of several plant-based brands and continues to consult with global grocery retailers, restaurants, and manufacturers on how to roll out healthy, sexy, plant-based foods to their customers.

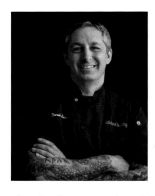

DEREK SARNO is the executive chef and director of plant-based innovation for Tesco, the third-largest food retailer in the world. Derek is cofounder of the Wicked Kitchen line of foods in Tesco and cofounder of Good Catch Foods. He is also the former senior global executive chef at Whole Foods Market, where he catered all of the company's major executive leadership events and oversaw national recipe development. After culinary school, Derek owned several critically acclaimed restaurants and catering businesses. He spent a few years farming and spent some quality time learning to meditate and cook a variety of foods at a Tibetan Buddhist monastery. Derek has always loved to train squirrels in the ways of the ninja. ←

FOR REAL!

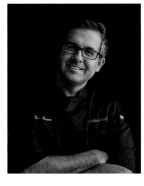

CHAD SARNO is vice president of culinary at Good Catch Foods and cofounder of the Wicked Kitchen line of foods in Tesco. Chad also is an ambassador for Rouxbe, the world's largest online cooking school, where he launched the Professional Plant-Based Certification course. He spent several years at Whole Foods Market as senior culinary educator and media spokesperson for the Global Healthy Eating program. Before that, Chad launched a line of boutique restaurants in Istanbul, Munich, and London. He has been a contributing author to more than a dozen cookbooks, and if not in the kitchen he's getting lost in his gardens.

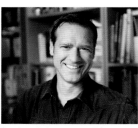

(credit: Olaf Starorypinski)

DAVID JOACHIM has authored, co-authored, or collaborated on more than forty cookbooks, including several award winners and bestsellers such as *The Food Substitutions Bible* and *A Man, a Can, a Plan*, a series of healthy cookbooks that has sold more than 1 million copies. He has been developing recipes for *Whole Foods Market* magazine since 2011 and co-writes a long-running column on food science in *Fine Cooking* magazine. He is the cofounder of Chef Salt artisan salt seasonings, and his favorite cooking tool is a leaf blower.